CROCKPOT COOKBOOK

Quick and Easy Recipes for Healthy Slow Cooker Meals

(Easy Crockpot Recipes for Busy Families)

Patricia Ross

Published by Alex Howard

© Patricia Ross

All Rights Reserved

Crockpot Cookbook: Quick and Easy Recipes for Healthy Slow Cooker Meals (Easy Crockpot Recipes for Busy Families)

ISBN 978-1-990169-93-9

All rights reserved. No part of this guide may be reproduced in any form without permission in writing from the publisher except in the case of brief quotations embodied in critical articles or reviews.

Legal & Disclaimer

The information contained in this book is not designed to replace or take the place of any form of medicine or professional medical advice. The information in this book has been provided for educational and entertainment purposes only.

The information contained in this book has been compiled from sources deemed reliable, and it is accurate to the best of the Author's knowledge; however, the Author cannot guarantee its accuracy and validity and cannot be held liable for any errors or omissions. Changes are periodically made to this book. You must consult your doctor or get professional medical advice before using any of the suggested remedies, techniques, or information in this book.

Table of contents

Part 1 1

Introductions.. 2

Chapter 1 – Crockpot Breakfast Options............................... 4

Recipe #1 – Spicy Peanut Butter Soup................................. 4

Recipe #2 – Marbled Tea Eggs with Brown Rice 5

Recipe #3 - Sweet Potato Soup with Cilantro and Cheese... 6

Recipe #4 – Coconut Curry Sauce with Noodles.................. 7

Recipe #5 – Rice and Chicken Soup..................................... 9

Slow Cooker Congee Recipes 10

Recipe #6 – Beef Quinoa Congee with Eggs 10

Recipe #7 - Beef Steak Congee with Olives and Peas..........12

Recipe #8 – Cauliflower and Seafood Quinoa Congee 14

Recipe #9 – Chicken and Cauliflower Quinoa Congee 16

Recipe #10 – Chicken and Corn Congee 18

Recipe #11 – Quail Eggs and Shallot Quinoa Congee 20

Recipe #12 - Sweet Coconut Congee.................................. 22

Recipe #13 – Tuna Congee with Corn and Peas 23

Slow Cooker Porridges Recipes 24

Recipe #14 - Almond Lake with Mandarin Oranges 24

Recipe #15 - Bacon and Cheese Porridge........................... 26

Recipe #16 – Banana and Blueberries Porridge.................28

Recipe #17 – Plain Banana Porridge 29

Recipe #18 – Banana and Pomegranate Porridge............. 30

Recipe #19 – Porridge with Nuts, Seeds, and Berries........ 31

Recipe #20 – Mushroom and Thyme Oatmeal 32

Recipe #21 – Peanut Oatmeal with Pork 33

Recipe #22 - Pork and Mushroom Porridge....................... 34

Recipe #23 – Unsalted Pistachio Porridge 36

Recipe #24 – Walnut Porridge with Strawberries 37

Recipe #25 – Oatmeal with Poached Egg 38

Chapter 2 – Crockpot Lunch Recipes................................... 40

Recipe #26 – Chicken and Egg Soup 40

Recipe #27 – Spaghetti Squash and Meatballs 41

Recipe #28 – Slow-Cooked Tilapia 43

Recipe #29 – Rolled Salmon... 44

Recipe #30 – Mustard Pork.. 45

Recipe #31 – Slow-Cooked Veggie Stew 46

Recipe #32 – Slow-Cooked Seitan Stew............................. 48

Recipe #33 – Spicy Quinoa 50

Recipe #34 – Slow-Cooked Eggplant 51

Recipe #35 – Chicken Asparagus 52

Recipe #36 – Chicken Mushroom 53

Recipe #37 – Chickpea Rice.. 55

Recipe #38 – Rice Enchilada 56

Recipe #39 – French Beans and Walnuts 57

Recipe #40 – Gumbo á La Louisiana 58

Recipe #41 – Seitan Brisket 60

Recipe #42 – Chili Tofu 61

Recipe #43 – Chickpea Curry 62

Recipe# 44 – White Bean and Sweet Potato Chili 64

Recipe #45 - Millet with Green Peas and Asparagus 66

Recipe #46 – Ginger Broccoli 67

Recipe #47 – Soyrizo and Beans 68

Recipe #48 – Veggie and Hulled Barley Medley 70

Recipe #49 – Vegetarian Chili 72

Recipe #50 – Stuffed Peppers with Wild Rice and Mushrooms 74

Chapter 3 – Delicious Homemade Slow Cooker Condiments 75

Fruit Jam Recipes 75

Recipe #51 - Balsamic Apricot Jam 75

Recipe #52 – Balsamic Blackberry Jam 76

Recipe #53 – Balsamic Cranberry Jam 77

Recipe #54 – 21 Balsamic Strawberry Jam 78

Recipe #55 – Blueberry and Raspberry Jam 79

Recipe #56 – Blackberry and Strawberry Jam 80

Recipe #57 – Chia Seeds Blueberry Jam 81

Recipe #58 – Apricot Jam..82

Recipe #59 – Cinnamon Apricot Jam.................................83

Recipe #60 – Blueberry Jam 84

Recipe #61 – Easy Mango Jam 85

Recipe #62 – Cinnamon Cranberry Jam 86

Recipe #63 – Blackberry Jam 87

Recipe #64 – Cherry Jam...88

Recipe #65 – Pineapple Jam..89

Recipe #66 – Peach Jam 90

Recipe #67 – Raspberry Jam 91

Recipe #68 – Plum Jam 92

Recipe #69 – Berry Jam...93

Recipe #70 – Strawberry Jam 94

Recipe #71 – Basil-Pumpkin Pesto Sauce...........................95

Recipe #72 – Basil-Walnut Pesto Sauce 96

Recipe #73 – Tomato Pesto Sauce...................................... 97

Recipe #74 – Cilantro Pesto Sauce.....................................98

Recipe #75 – Cilantro-Cashew Pesto Sauce......................99

Recipe #76 – Cilantro-Walnut Pesto Sauce..................... 100

Recipe #77 – Kale Pesto Sauce 101

Recipe #78 – Kale-Cashew Pesto Sauce.......................... 102

Recipe #79 – Kale-Walnut Pesto Sauce 103

Recipe #80 – Mint Pesto Sauce.. 104

Chapter 4 – Crockpot Dinner Selections 105

Recipe #81 – Coconut and Ginger Linguine..................... 105

Recipe #82 – Vegan Mac 'n' Cheese................................... 107

Recipe #83 – Barley and Butternut Squash Casserole 108

Recipe #84 – Seitan in Soy Yogurt..................................... 109

Recipe #85 – Yummy Glazed Salmon 110

Recipe #86 – Cranberry-Apple Pork................................... 111

Recipe #87 – Herbed Tenderloin 112

Recipe #88 – Guilt-Free Stroganoff....................................113

Recipe #89 – Slow-Cooked Rice and Bean Dish 114

Recipe #90 – Corn and Mushroom.....................................115

Recipe #91 – Three Bean Chili..116

Recipe #92 – Butternut Squash and Beef Stew.................117

Recipe #93 – Sweet Corn-Bean-Beef Chili 118

Recipe #94 – Veggie Curry..119

Recipe #95 – Tasty Farfelle.. 120

Recipe #96 – Scrumptious Lentil Soup 121

Recipe #97 – Pumpkin Soup.. 122

Recipe #98 – Savory Roasted Cabbage............................. 123

Recipe #99 – Thai Tofu Bowls... 124

Recipe #100 – Sweet Potato and Beef............................... 126

Conclusion 127

Part 2 128

BEEF RECIPES 129

Crock Pot Beef Stew 129

Our Go-To Recipe for Shredded Beef 132

Slow Cooked Shredded Spicy Beef 133

Roasted Garlic and Brown Sugar Pulled Roast Sandwiches 135

Crock Pot Swiss Steak 137

Easy Corned Beef and Cabbage 139

Easy Pepper Steak 142

Delicious Balsamic and Worcestershire Roast Beef 144

Mouthwatering Beef Nachos with Fresh Pico de Gallo 146

Roast Beef with Pineapple 148

Slow Cooker Cheeseburgers 150

Tender Coconut Curry Vegetables and Beef 152

Easy Slow Cooker Meatballs 154

Lighter Beef and Mushroom Stroganoff 156

CHICKEN RECIPES 158

Slow Cooked Lime and Cilantro Chicken 158

Crock Pot Lemon Chicken with Baby Carrots 160

Crock Pot Marinara Vegetables with Chicken 162

Tender Herbed Chicken 163

Sweet Potato, Mushroom, and Chicken Stew 166

Cashew Chicken 167

Crock Pot Wild Rice and Chicken Stew 169

Slow Cooker Taco Soup with Chicken 171

Crock Pot Creamy Chicken Stroganoff 173

Cheesy Slow Cooker Chicken & Rice 176

Juicy Crock Pot Chicken Marbella 177

Garlic and Cinnamon Slow Cooked Chicken 179

Spicy Chorizo Chicken 181

Slow Cooker Chicken and Dumplings 183

Delicious Mexican Chicken Tortilla Soup 184

Part 1

Introductions

Slow cookers or crockpots have become our best tools in the recent years because it allows us to a) put everything into the slow cooker, b) allow meals to prepare itself, and c) saves money, time, and efforts. Gone are the days of time-consuming and tedious work in the kitchen just to prepare for the day's meals. You have gone through hours waiting in line at the grocery, and cooking for an hour or two just don't do justice. Good thing, there are slow cookers to do the job for you. If this sounds good to you, then this quick and easy recipes cookbook is for you.

With a slow cooker, all you need is just few minutes to prepare the ingredients and then you can just leave it and attend to your other chores. If the recipe calls for some frying before dumping all ingredients into the slow cooker or processing after, it won't take you 10 minutes to do it.

The very idea of a slow cooker is to cook dishes slowly at a stable temperature. So even if it is turned on for more than 8 hours, it still has the same electric consumption as that of your regular lightbulb. Slow cookers are economical and are easy on the pocket.

This cookbook presents **100 crockpot recipes** that you can easily prepare in minutes and wait for the slow cooker to do its magic. The recipes you will find here are divided into 4 categories: breakfast, lunch, condiments, and dinner.

All you need is to grab a good Crockpot or Slow Cooker if you don't already have one kicking around in your home to get started today to prepare crockpot cooked, easy and healthy recipes for your meals. I am sure you will find some amazing quick and easy recipes in this cookbook with little efforts.

Chapter 1 – Crockpot Breakfast Options

Recipe #1 – Spicy Peanut Butter Soup

Ingredients:

- 4 cups unsalted mushroom stock
- ½ cup organic peanut butter
- 2 pieces large minced garlic cloves
- 2 pieces large minced yellow onion
- 1 piece, large acorn squash, peeled, deseeded, cubed
- 1 piece, large green Serrano pepper, deseeded, minced
- 1 Tbsp. olive oil
- 1 Tbsp. fresh ginger, peeled, grated
- Salt
- White pepper

Directions:

1. Pour oil into non-stick pot set over medium heat. When oil is hot enough, add in and sauté onion and garlic until limp and aromatic. Add in remaining ingredients. Stir.
2. Transfer to the slow cooker. Cover the lid and cook for 4 hours on low.
3. Cool before processing into a blender until smooth. Taste; adjust seasoning, if needed. Ladle recommended portion into bowls and serve.

Recipe #2 – Marbled Tea Eggs with Brown Rice

Ingredients:

- 4 large eggs, soft-boiled, using back of spoon, lightly crack shells to produce marbling effect
- 2 cups brown rice, cooked according to package instructions, divided into 4 equal portions, kept warm

Marinade

- 1 piece star anise
- 1 cup water
- ¼ cup light soy sauce
- ¼ cup brown sugar
- ½ Tbsp. loose leaf smoked tea, preferably black tea
- ¼ Tbsp. fennel seeds
- ¼ Tbsp. whole black peppercorns
- ⅛ Tbsp. cinnamon powder
- sea salt to taste

Directions:

1. Except for tea leaves, place marinade ingredients into slow cooker. Cover the lid and cook for 4 hours on low. Add in tea leaves and cracked eggs; steep for 15 minutes or longer. Drain and discard marinade. Peel eggs when cool enough.
2. Place equal portions of brown rice into bowls. Place marbled egg in the middle. Serve with dash of sea salt if using.

Recipe #3 - Sweet Potato Soup with Cilantro and Cheese

Ingredients:

- 4 cups unsalted mushroom stock
- 2 cans, 15 oz. sweet potato puree
- 1 Tbsp. olive oil
- 1 piece, large garlic cloves, peeled, minced
- 1 piece, large white onion, peeled, minced
- Salt
- Mixed dry or fresh herbs
- White pepper

For garnish

- ¼ cup macadamia nut cheese with olives, divided
- ¼ cup chopped fresh cilantro

Directions:

1. Pour oil into a pot set over medium heat. When oil is hot enough, add in and sauté onion and garlic until limp and aromatic. Transfer into the slow cooker.
2. Except for garnishes, add in remaining ingredients. Stir. Cover the lid and cook for 6 hours on low.
3. Cool slightly before processing into a blender until smooth. Taste; adjust seasoning, if needed. Ladle into bowls. Add equal portions of garnishes on top.

Recipe #4 – Coconut Curry Sauce with Noodles

Ingredients:

For the noodles
- 2 green courgettes
- 1 large carrot
- 2 yellow courgettes
- 2 corn cobs kernels
- 1 large handful mixed herbs
- 200 grams fresh peas

For the sauce

- 1 banana shallot
- 2 tsps. ground turmeric
- 1 garlic clove
- 1 lime
- 300 ml coconut water
- 200 ml coconut milk
- 1 tsp. hot curry powder
- 100g desiccated unsweetened coconut

Directions:
1. Remove the skin from the ginger, garlic, and shallot and roughly chop. Take the zest and juice from the lime.
2. Add the shallot, turmeric, garlic, lime zest, lime juice, coconut water, coconut milk, curry powder, and coconut in a food processor. Process until the creamy and smooth. Transfer into the slow cooker. Cover the lid and cook for 2 hours on low.

3. Using a spiralizer or a julienne peeler, turn the carrot and courgettes into vegetable noodles.
4. Place the vegetable noodles in a salad bowl together with the corn, mixed herbs, and peas. Pour over the sauce and toss until well-coated. Set aside for 30 minutes. Squeeze extra lime on top before serving.

Recipe #5 – Rice and Chicken Soup

Ingredients:
- 1 cup sliced mushrooms
- 1 chopped onion
- ½ cup uncooked rice
- 2 sliced celery ribs
- 4 cups low or no sodium and fat-free chicken broth
- 2 medium carrots halved
- 1 cup sliced green beans
- 2 cups of cooked chopped chicken breast

Directions:
1. Pour the broth into the slow cooker. Add the rice and vegetables. Cover the lid and cook for 4 hours on low.
2. Stir in the cooked chicken. Reposition the lid. Cover and cook on low for another 1 hour. Serve.

Slow Cooker Congee Recipes

Congee is a staple in Chinese cuisine, and is gradually becoming one in many American homes, too. Though this is often served for breakfast, you can also serve congee for lunch or dinner as well. To save time, prepare dishes the night before. Set your slow cooker at the recommended time, and leave it to cook on its own. Your meals will remain warm next day.

Or, if you are making these for dinner, prep your dishes before you leave the house in the morning. If desired, cook and freeze large batches, and reheat a serving or two in the microwave as needed.

Recipe #6 – Beef Quinoa Congee with Eggs

Ingredients:

- 6 cups water
- ½ cup red quinoa
- 2 pieces grated large garlic cloves
- Mince 2 pieces large leeks and keep some for garnish
- 1 Tbsp. coconut oil
- 1 Tbsp. red rice, rinsed, drained
- ½ Tbsp. dark low sodium soy sauce
- ¼ Tbsp. fish sauce
- ½ tsp. grated ginger
- ⅛ tsp. white pepper to taste
- ¼ pound extra lean ground beef
- Mixed dry or fresh herbs
- Salt and pepper

Garnishes

- 2 large eggs, boiled, peeled, quartered lengthwise, substitute boiled chicken eggs if desired
- Dash of red pepper flakes
- Dash of garlic flakes

Directions:

1. Pour oil into non-stick skillet set over medium heat. Sauté leeks and garlic until limp and aromatic; add in beef. Stir-fry until meat browns; add the herbs; and pour into slow cooker set at medium heat.
2. Except for garnishes, pour in remaining ingredients; stir. Put lid on. Cook for 6 hours. Turn off heat. Taste; adjust seasoning if needed.
3. Ladle congee into individual bowls. Garnish with leeks and century eggs. Sprinkle in garlic flakes and red pepper flakes. Cool slightly before serving.

Recipe #7 - Beef Steak Congee with Olives and Peas

Ingredients:

- 6 cups water
- ¼ cup brown or red rice (rinsed and drained)
- ¼ cup frozen corn, thawed, drained
- ¼ cup frozen peas, thawed, drained
- 2 pieces grated large garlic cloves
- 2 pieces large black olives in brine, rinsed, drained, pitted, roughly chopped
- 1 piece large shallot, minced
- 1 Tbsp. coconut oil
- ½ Tbsp. fish sauce
- ½ pound beef hanger steak, diced
- Salt
- Mixed dry or fresh herbs
- Black pepper to taste

Garnishes

- 1 piece small lime, sliced into wedges, pips removed
- ⅛ cup fresh minced chives

Directions:

1. Pour oil into non-stick skillet set over medium heat. Sauté garlic and shallots until limp and aromatic; add in beef; and add herbs.
2. Stir-fry until meat browns; pour into slow cooker set at high heat. Except for garnishes, pour in remaining

ingredients; stir. Put lid on. Cook for 6 hours. Turn off heat. Taste; adjust seasoning if needed.
3. Ladle congee into individual bowls. Garnish with equal portions of chives. Serve with wedge of lime. Squeeze lime juice over congee just before eating.

Recipe #8 – Cauliflower and Seafood Quinoa Congee

Ingredients:

- 6 cups water
- ¼ cup quinoa
- 4 pieces large leeks, roots removed, minced, reserve green stems for garnish
- 1 piece small cauliflower head, minced
- 1 can 5 oz. mackerel in water, low-sodium, include liquid, flaked
- 1 Tbsp. fresh ginger, grated
- 1 Tbsp. fish sauce, add more later only if needed
- ¼ pound frozen scallops, thawed, blanched, drained
- ¼ pound frozen shrimps, thawed, blanched, drained
- Salt
- Mixed dry or fresh herbs
- White pepper to taste

Garnishes

- 4 slivers large smoked salmon, roughly torn, optional
- 1 piece small lime, sliced into wedges, pips removed

Directions:

1. Except for garnishes, scallops, and shrimps, pour remaining ingredients into slow cooker set at low heat. Stir. Put lid on.

2. Cook for 6 hours. Stir in scallops and shrimps; cook for another 15 minutes. Turn off heat. Taste; adjust seasoning if needed.
3. Ladle congee into individual bowls. Garnish with leeks and smoked salmon if using. Serve with wedge of lime on the side. Squeeze lime juice into congee just before eating.

Recipe #9 – Chicken and Cauliflower Quinoa Congee

Ingredients:

- 6 cups water
- 2 Tbsp. heaping red quinoa
- 2 Tbsp. heaping red rice, rinsed, drained
- 1 Tbsp. coconut oil
- 1 Tbsp. fresh grated ginger
- 1 Tbsp. fish sauce, add more later only if needed
- 2 pieces large chicken thigh fillets, minced
- 2 pieces large leeks, roots removed, minced
- 2 pieces large shallots, minced
- 2 pieces large garlic cloves, grated
- 1 piece small cauliflower head, minced
- Salt
- Mixed dry or fresh herbs
- white pepper to taste

Garnishes

- 4 pieces extra small chicken eggs, soft-boiled, peeled
- 2 pieces large red chili, deseeded, minced
- 1 piece small lime, sliced into wedges, pips removed
- ¼ cup loosely packed Asian basil leaves, rinsed, drained, torn
- ¼ cup loosely packed cilantro leaves, rinsed, drained, torn
- ¼ cup loosely packed spearmint leaves, rinsed, drained, torn

Directions:

1. Pour oil into large skillet set over medium heat. Sauté shallots, garlic, and ginger until limp and aromatic; pour into slow cooker set at medium heat.
2. Except for garnishes, pour remaining ingredients into slow cooker; stir. Put lid on. Cook for 6 hours. Turn off heat. Taste; adjust seasoning if needed.
3. Ladle congee into individual bowls. Garnish with basil leaves, cilantro leaves, red chili, and spearmint leaves. Add 1 piece of soft-boiled chicken egg on top of each; serve with wedge of lime on the side.
4. Slice egg just before eating so yolk runs into congee. Squeeze lime juice into congee just before eating.

Recipe #10 – Chicken and Corn Congee

Ingredients:

- 6 cups water
- ¼ cup brown or red rice, rinsed, drained
- ¼ cup frozen corn, thawed, drained
- 2 pieces large garlic cloves, grated
- 1 piece large shallot, minced
- 1 piece thumb-sized ginger, peeled, crushed using flat side of knife
- 1 Tbsp. coconut oil
- 1 Tbsp. fish sauce
- ½ pound chicken thigh fillets, diced
- Mixed dry or fresh herbs
- Salt
- Black pepper to taste

Garnishes

- 1 piece small lime, sliced into wedges, pips removed
- ⅛ cup fresh cilantro, minced
- Dash of garlic flakes

Directions:

1. Pour oil into non-stick skillet set over medium heat. Sauté garlic and shallots until limp and aromatic; add in chicken. Stir-fry until meat browns; add mix herbs and pour into slow cooker set at medium heat.
2. Except for garnishes, pour in remaining ingredients; stir. Put lid on. Cook for 6 hours. Turn off heat. Fish out and discard ginger. Taste; adjust seasoning if needed.

3. Ladle congee into individual bowls. Garnish with equal portions of cilantro and garlic flakes. Serve with wedge of lime. Squeeze lime juice over congee just before eating.

Recipe #11 – Quail Eggs and Shallot Quinoa Congee

Ingredients:

- 8 pieces quail eggs, hardboiled, peeled, halved
- 2 pieces large shallots, julienned
- 1 piece large chicken egg, whisked
- 1 piece small lime, sliced into wedges, pips removed, for garnish
- 3 cups chicken or vegetable stock, low-sodium
- 3 cups water
- ¼ cup quinoa
- 2 Tbsp. garlic flakes
- 2 Tbsp. coconut oil
- 1 Tbsp. fish sauce, add more later only if needed
- Salt
- Mixed dry or fresh herbs
- White pepper to taste

Directions:

1. Pour oil into large skillet set over medium heat. Stir-fry shallots until toasted brown. Temporarily place crispy shallots into a bowl.
2. Toast quinoa in leftover oil until seeds give off a nut-like aroma. Pour this, along with chicken stock, fish sauce, and water into slow cooker set at low heat; stir.
3. Put lid on. Cook for 6 hours. Turn off heat. Except for lime and quail eggs, stir in remaining ingredients. Taste; adjust seasoning if needed.
4. Ladle congee into individual bowls. Garnish with quail eggs and crispy shallots on top. Serve with wedge of

lime on the side. Squeeze lime juice into congee just before eating.

Recipe #12 - Sweet Coconut Congee

Ingredients:

- 6 cups water
- ¼ cup brown rice
- ¼ cup ripe jackfruit, peeled, deseeded, shredded
- ¼ cup tapioca pearls, large pearls, cooked according to package instructions, drained
- ⅛ cup palm sugar, crumbled, reserve some for sprinkling
- 2 cans, 15 oz. coconut cream, divided
- 1 can, 15 oz. whole corn kernels, rinsed, drained
- Salt
- 1 piece, large fresh banana, thinly sliced, for garnish

Directions:

1. Except for banana, cooked tapioca pearls, and 1 can of coconut cream, pour remaining ingredients into slow cooker set at low heat.
2. Stir. Put lid on. Cook for 6 hours. Pour in remaining can of coconut cream and tapioca pearls; stir. Taste; adjust seasoning if needed.
3. Ladle congee into individual bowls. Garnish with equal portions of banana slices. Sprinkle more palm sugar on top. Cool slightly before serving.

Recipe #13 – Tuna Congee with Corn and Peas

Ingredients:

- 6 cups water
- ¼ cup brown or red rice, rinsed, drained
- ¼ cup frozen corn, thawed, drained
- ¼ cup frozen peas, thawed, drained
- 2 pieces large garlic cloves, grated
- 1 piece large shallot, minced
- 1 Tbsp. coconut oil
- 1 Tbsp. fish sauce
- 1 can, 5 oz. tuna chunks in brine, flaked
- ¼ tsp. fresh grated finger
- Salt
- Black pepper to taste

Garnishes

- 1 piece small lime, sliced into wedges, pips removed
- ⅛ cup fresh chives, minced

Directions:

1. Pour oil into large sauté pan set over medium heat. Sauté garlic and shallots until limp and aromatic; pour into slow cooker set at low heat.
2. Except for garnishes, pour in remaining ingredients; stir. Put lid on. Cook for 6 hours. Turn off heat. Taste; adjust seasoning if needed.
3. Ladle congee into individual bowls. Garnish with chives and serve wedge of lime on the side. Squeeze lime juice over congee just before eating.

Slow Cooker Porridges Recipes

Sweet and savory porridges are far better substitutes for sugary breakfast cereals. These recipes can fill you up in the morning despite being low in carbohydrates. Like congee recipes in this book, you can start these dishes the night before. Add remaining ingredients and garnishes when you are ready to serve.

Recipe #14 - Almond Lake with Mandarin Oranges

Ingredients:

- 3 cups water
- 1 cup unsweetened almond milk
- ¾ cup steel-cut oats, gluten-free if preferred
- 2 pieces large overripe bananas, mashed
- 1 drop almond extract
- 1 Tbsp., heaping almond slivers, fresh toasted on dry pan
- 1 can, 3.5 oz. mandarin oranges in light syrup, drained lightly, divided into 4 equal portions
- Brown sugar

Directions:

1. Pour steel cut oats and water in slow cooker set at low heat. Put lid on. Cook for 6 hours. Turn heat off. Stir in almond extract, almond milk, and bananas. Taste; add brown sugar only if needed.

2. Ladle equal portions of porridge into bowls. Garnish with almond slivers and mandarin oranges on top. Cool slightly before serving.

Recipe #15 - Bacon and Cheese Porridge

Ingredients:

- 8 slices large bacon, minced
- 4 Tbsp. water

For porridge

- 2 cups beef or vegetable no sodium stock
- 1 cup milk
- 1 cup water
- ¾ cup steel-cut oats, gluten-free if desired
- ½ cup cheddar cheese, grated
- 1 piece minced large shallot
- Salt
- Mixed herbs
- White pepper to taste

Garnishes

- ½ cup grape tomatoes, quartered
- ¼ cup fresh chives, minced

Directions:

1. Place bacon and water into non-stick skillet set over high heat. Stirring often, cook bacon bits until fat renders out and meat crisps; temporarily transfer cooked pieces to a small bowl.
2. In the same skillet, sauté shallot until limp and transparent; transfer contents into slow cooker set at low heat. Except for cheddar cheese and garnishes, pour remaining ingredients into slow cooker; stir.

3. Put lid on. Cook porridge for 6 hours. Stir in cheddar cheese. Taste; adjust seasoning if needed.
4. Ladle equal portions of porridge into individual bowls. Garnish with grape tomatoes and chives. Cool slightly before serving.

Recipe #16 – Banana and Blueberries Porridge

Ingredients:

- 4 cups water
- 1 cup raw cashew nuts, minced
- 1 cup fresh blueberries
- ¾ cup steel-cut oats, gluten-free if desired
- 2 pieces large overripe bananas, mashed
- Brown sugar, if needed

Directions:

1. Pour cashew nuts, steel cut oats and water in slow cooker set at low heat. Put lid on. Cook for 6 hours. Turn heat off. Stir in mashed bananas. Taste; add brown sugar only if needed.
2. Ladle equal portions of porridge into individual bowls. Garnish with fresh blueberries. Cool slightly before serving.

Recipe#17 – Plain Banana Porridge

Ingredients:

- 4 cups water
- ¾ cup steel-cut oats, gluten-free if desired
- 2 pieces large overripe bananas, mashed
- Brown sugar, only if needed, optional

Garnishes

- 2 Tbsp., heaping raw almonds, roughly chopped
- 2 Tbsp., heaping raw cashew nuts, roughly chopped
- 2 Tbsp., heaping raw walnuts, roughly chopped
- 2 Tbsp. dried goji berries
- 2 Tbsp. dried Inca berries
- 2 Tbsp. raisins

Directions:

1. Pour steel cut oats and water in slow cooker set at low heat. Put lid on. Cook for 6 hours. Turn heat off. Stir in mashed bananas. Taste; add brown sugar only if needed.
2. Toast almonds, cashew nuts and walnuts in non-stick skillet set over high heat until brown and aromatic.
3. Ladle equal portions of porridge into individual bowls. Garnish with toasted nuts, dried berries and raisins. Cool slightly before serving.

Recipe #18 – Banana and Pomegranate Porridge

Ingredients:

- 4 cups water
- ¾ cup steel-cut oats, gluten-free if desired
- 2 pieces large overripe bananas, mashed
- 1 piece large pomegranate, seeds whacked out, juices extracted
- Brown sugar, if needed

Directions:

1. Pour steel cut oats and water in slow cooker set at low heat. Put lid on. Cook for 6 hours. Turn heat off.
2. Stir in mashed bananas and pomegranate juice. Taste; add palm sugar only if needed.
3. Ladle equal portions of porridge into individual bowls. Garnish with pomegranate seeds. Cool slightly before serving.

Recipe #19 – Porridge with Nuts, Seeds, and Berries

Ingredients:

- 4 cups water
- ¾ cup steel-cut oats
- 2 pieces large overripe bananas, mashed
- Balm sugar, if needed

Garnishes

- 2 Tbsp. roasted cashew nuts, roughly chopped
- 2 Tbsp. roasted walnuts, roughly chopped
- ¼ tsp. caraway seeds, toasted on dry pan
- ¼ tsp. chia seeds, toasted on dry pan
- 1 cup heaping fresh strawberries, hulled
- ½ cup fresh blackberries
- ½ cup fresh blueberries

Directions:

1. Pour steel cut oats and water in slow cooker set at low heat. Put lid on. Cook for 6 hours. Turn heat off. Stir in mashed bananas. Taste; add brown sugar only if needed.
2. Ladle equal portions porridge into individual bowls. Garnish with toasted nuts and seeds. Add generous portions of fresh berries. Serve.

Recipe #20 – Mushroom and Thyme Oatmeal

Ingredients:

- 4 cups water
- ¾ cup steel-cut oats, gluten-free if desired
- ½ cup smoked grated Gouda cheese
- 2 sprigs fresh whole thyme
- 2 Tbsp. coconut oil
- 2 pieces large minced garlic cloves
- 1 piece large julienned onion
    - ¼ pound fresh button mushrooms, cleaned well using paper towels, julienned
- Salt
- Mixed herbs
- White pepper to taste

Directions:

1. Pour 1 Tbsp. of oil into large skillet set over medium heat. Fry mushrooms until golden brown on all sides. Push to one side of skillet. Pour in remaining oil; sauté garlic and onion until limp and aromatic. Mix with mushrooms; add mix herbs; and pour into slow cooker set at low heat.
2. Except for smoked Gouda, pour remaining ingredients into slow cooker; stir. Put lid on. Cook for 6 hours. Turn off heat. Fish out and discard thyme. Stir in Gouda cheese. Taste; adjust seasoning if needed.
3. Ladle equal portions of porridge into individual bowls. Serve.

Recipe #21 – Peanut Oatmeal with Pork

Ingredients:

- 2 cups mushroom or vegetable unsalted stock
- 2 cups water
- ¾ cup steel-cut oats, gluten-free if desired
- ½ cup, loosely packed pork floss, shredded
- 2 pieces large garlic clove, minced
- 1 piece large shallot, minced
- 1 tsp. fresh ginger, grated
- Salt
- White pepper to taste

Garnishes

- 2 Tbsp. garlic-roasted peanuts, roughly chopped
- 1 tsp. black sesame seeds, toasted on dry pan
- 1 piece large Serrano chili, deseeded, minced

Directions:

1. Except for garnishes, pour ingredients into slow cooker set over low heat, add salt. Put lid on. Cook for 6 hours. Stir. Taste; adjust seasoning if needed.
2. Ladle equal portions of porridge into bowls. Garnish with chili, peanuts, and sesame seeds. Serve.

Recipe #22 - Pork and Mushroom Porridge

Ingredients:

- 3 cups pork or mushroom no or low sodium stock
- 3 cups water
- ¾ cup millet, rinsed, drained
- 2 Tbsp. olive oil, add more only if needed
- 1 Tbsp. light low sodium soy sauce
- ¼ Tbsp. fish sauce, add more later if desired
- 2 pieces large minced garlic clove
- 1 piece large minced shallot
- ¼ pound fresh shiitake mushrooms, cleaned using paper towels, tough parts removed, sliced into ⅛-inch thick slivers
- ¼ pound lean pork shoulder, diced
- ½ tsp. fresh minced ginger
- Mixed herbs
- White pepper to taste

Garnishes

- ¼ cup, loosely packed fresh chives, minced
- ¼ cup, packed pork cracklings, crushed
- 1 tsp. garlic flakes
- Drops chili oil

Directions:

1. Pour oil into large non-stick skillet set over medium heat. Stir-fry shiitake mushrooms until golden brown on all sides, adding more oil as needed. Transfer cooked pieces into slow cooker. Pour a little more oil into skillet; sauté garlic, ginger, mixed herbs, and shallot until limp and aromatic.

2. Add in diced pork; stir-fry until meat loses its pinkness. Transfer contents of skillet into slow cooker set at medium heat.
3. Except for garnishes, pour in remaining ingredients; stir. Put lid on. Cook for 6 hours. Turn off heat. Taste; adjust seasoning if needed.
4. Ladle equal portions of porridge into bowls. Garnish with chives, cracklings, and garlic flakes. Add a drop of two of chili oil for heat. Cool slightly before serving.

Recipe #23 – Unsalted Pistachio Porridge

Ingredients:

- 4 cups water
- ¾ cup millet, rinsed, drained
- ¼ cup shelled, roasted pistachio nuts, roughly chopped, for garnish
- 2 cans. 15 oz. each coconut cream, divided
- 2 pieces, large overripe bananas, mashed
- 1 piece, large mango, peeled, pitted, diced
- Brown sugar, crumbled, only if needed

Directions:

1. Pour millet, water and 1 can of coconut cream into slow cooker set at low heat. Stir. Put lid on. Cook for 6 hours. Turn off heat. Except for pistachio nuts, stir in remaining ingredients.
2. Ladle equal portions of porridge into bowls. Garnish with pistachio nuts. Cool slightly before serving.

Recipe #24 – Walnut Porridge with Strawberries

Ingredients:

- 4 cups water
- 2 cups, heaping fresh strawberries, hulled, quartered
- ¾ cup millet, rinsed, drained
- ¼ cup roasted walnuts, chopped, for garnish
- 2 cans 15 oz. each coconut cream, divided
- 2 pieces, large overripe bananas, mashed
- Brown sugar, crumbled, only if needed

Directions:

1. Pour millet, water and 1 can of coconut cream into slow cooker set at low heat. Stir. Put lid on. Cook for 6 hours. Turn off heat.
2. Except for walnuts, stir in remaining ingredients.
3. Ladle equal portions of porridge into bowls. Garnish with walnuts. Cool slightly before serving.

Recipe #25 – Oatmeal with Poached Egg

Ingredients:

- 4 pieces of large leeks, minced
- 2 cups mushroom or vegetable stock, unsalted
- 2 cups water
- ¾ cup steel-cut oats, gluten-free if desired
- 1 Tbsp. coconut oil
- 1 Tbsp. light soy sauce
- 1 tsp. fresh ginger, grated
- ¼ pound fresh button mushrooms, cleaned well using paper towels, minced
- Salt
- White pepper to taste

Garnishes, divided

- 4 precut pieces, 2"x2" each dried wakame seaweed, substitute *nori* or *kombu* if desired
    - 4 pieces, extra small poached chicken eggs, substitute peeled soft-boiled eggs if desired
- 1 piece, small lime, sliced into wedges, pips removed
- ¼ cup, loosely packed bean sprouts, rinsed, drained well
- ¼ cup, loosely packed fresh baby spinach, roughly torn
- ¼ cup, loosely packed fresh basil leaves, roughly torn
- ¼ cup, loosely packed fresh cilantro, roughly torn

Directions:

1. Pour oil into large non-stick skillet set over medium heat. Stir-fry button mushrooms until golden brown on all sides; transfer into slow cooker set at low heat.
2. Except for garnishes, pour in remaining ingredients into slow cooker. Put lid on. Cook for 6 hours. Stir. Taste; adjust seasoning if needed.
3. Place a piece of dried wakame into each bowl; ladle equal portions of porridge on top.
4. Garnish with bean sprouts, baby spinach, basil leaves and cilantro; add poached eggs in the middle of herbs. Serve with wedge of lime. Squeeze lime into porridge just before eating.

Chapter 2 – Crockpot Lunch Recipes

Recipe #26 – Chicken and Egg Soup

Ingredients:
- ½ cup mushrooms, finely chopped
- ½ cup onion, finely chopped
- ¼ cup ketchup, tomato
- ½ cup carrots, grated
- 1 tablespoon sauce, Worcestershire
- 1 pound chicken, ground, extra-lean
- ¼ cup parsley, fresh, finely chopped
- ½ cup breadcrumbs, dried
- 1 egg, large, beaten lightly

Directions:
1. Place the mushrooms, ground chicken, carrots, parsley, and onion in a large mixing bowl. Combine the ingredients before stirring in the egg, ketchup, and Worcestershire sauce.
2. Transfer into the slow cooker. Cover the lid and cook for 4 hours on low. Adjust taste. Serve

Recipe #27 – Spaghetti Squash and Meatballs

Ingredients:
- 2 spaghetti squash
- 1 cup marinara sauce
- 1 lb ground turkey
- 1 cup shredded mozzarella cheese
- Olive oil
- 1 zucchini
- 1.2 onion, chopped
- 1 egg white
- Sea salt
- Ground black pepper, to taste
- 1 tbsp. Worcestershire sauce
- 4 garlic cloves
- ½ cup almond flour
- 5 oz mozzarella cheese
- 1 cup marinara sauce
- ½ teaspoon Italian seasoning

Directions:
1. In a food processor, grate onion, garlic and zucchini. Add egg white, Italian seasoning, almond flour, Worcestershire sauce, turkey, salt and pepper to the food processor and pulse to combine all the ingredients together.

2. Shape mixture into meatballs. Each meatball is about two tablespoons of the turkey mixture.
3. Transfer meatballs and marinara sauce into the slow cooker. Cover the lid and cook for 6 hours on low.
4. Take spaghetti squash and pierce it on all sides with a small knife up to its center. Microwave squash for 3 minutes.
5. Cut squash in half and remove the seeds. Lay the squash on a greased baking sheet lined with foil. Season with salt and pepper. Roast squash in the oven for 1 hour or until fully tender.
6. Allow squash to cool. Scrape the inside of the squash to fluff up the flesh. Take meatballs out of the slow cooker. Top with meatballs marinara sauce and mozzarella cheese.

Recipe #28 – Slow-Cooked Tilapia

Ingredients:
- 2 tsps. ground cumin
- 4 fillets, tilapia, five-ounce
- 1 tsps cheese, reduced-fat, shredded
- 14 ½ oz tomatoes, Mexican-style

Directions:
1. Arrange the tilapia fillets inside the slow cooker. Lightly coat the fillets with black pepper and cumin. Pour in tomatoes.
2. Cover the lid and cook for 8 on low or 4 hours on high. Top with cheese before serving.

Recipe #29 – Rolled Salmon

Ingredients:
- 4 oz cream cheese, fat-free
- 4 oz salmon, smoked, thinly sliced
- Lemon wedge
- ½ tsp. freshly ground black pepper
- 1 bag arugula leaves

Directions:
1. Put smoked salmon slices inside the slow cooker. Sprinkle with pepper before rolling up each slice. Cover the lid and cook for 4 hours on high.
2. Take salmon out of the slow cooker. Slice salmon rolls into half-inch portions. Sprinkle with cheese. Place in the refrigerator for 1 hour.
3. Serve salmon rolls on a large platter with lemon wedges and arugula leaves.

Recipe #30 – Mustard Pork

Ingredients:
- 1 medium shallot, finely chopped
- 1 tbsp. Dijon mustard
- 1/3 cup white wine, dry
- 3/4 pound pork tenderloin
- 8 ounces mushrooms, sliced
- 1 tbsp. flour
- ¾ cup chicken broth, low-sodium, fat-free
- 1 tbsp. olive oil

Directions:
1. Cut trimmed tenderloin into eight rounds. Flatten pork medallions before placing inside the slow cooker. Sprinkle with salt and pepper. Add mushrooms and shallots. Pour in broth and mustard. Stir well to combine.
2. Cover the lid. Cook for 4 hours on low. Take the pork out of the slow cooker. Serve right away.

Recipe #31 – Slow-Cooked Veggie Stew

Ingredients:
- 1 tbsp. olive oil
- 2 minced garlic clove
- 1 onion, diced
- 1 large carrot, chopped
- 1 oz cremini mushrooms, sliced
- 1 lb sweet potatoes, diced
- 2 ½ tbsps. whole wheat flour
- 1/3 cup water
- 1 ½ tbsps. tomato paste
- 2 cups vegetable broth
- 1 cup red wine
- ½ tsp. dried rosemary
- ½ tsp. dried thyme
- ½ tsp. paprika
- ½ tsp. fennel, crushed
- Salt
- Ground black pepper, to taste

Directions:
1. Combine olive oil, garlic clove, onion, carrot, cremini mushrooms, sweet potatoes, flour, water, tomato paste, vegetable broth, red wine, rosemary, thyme, paprika, and fennel in the slow cooker. Mix well. Season to taste with salt and pepper.

2. Cover and cook on low for 6 hours, stirring once every few hours. Best served warm.

Recipe #32 – Slow-Cooked Seitan Stew

Ingredients:
- 1 ½ tbsps. olive oil
- 1 ½ lb seitan, cubed
- 8 oz canned diced tomatoes, juices reserved
- 2 garlic cloves
- 1 cup celery, chopped
- ½ tsp sea salt
- 1/8 tsp freshly ground black pepper
- 1/4 cup dry red wine

For the Spice Blend:
- 1/8 tsp ground cloves
- 1/8 tsp ground cinnamon
- Ground nutmeg
- Ground allspice

Directions:
1. Mix together spice blend ingredients. Set aside.
2. Put seitan in the slow cooker. Add garlic and celery. Season with salt, spice blend, and diced tomatoes with their juices. Pour wine and stir well to combine.
3. Cover and cook on low for 4 hours. Transfer to a serving dish and serve right away.

Recipe #33 – Spicy Quinoa

Ingredients:
- ½ cup quinoa, rinsed thoroughly
- ½ cup water
- 14 oz kidney beans, drained and rinsed
- 1 cup diced tomatoes
- 8 z black beans, drained and rinsed
- 1 cup frozen corn kernels, thawed
- 1 ½ tablespoons olive oil
- ½ small onion, diced
- ½ red bell pepper, diced
- 2 garlic cloves
- 2 teaspoons cumin
- 1 ½ teaspoons dried oregano
- 1 teaspoon chili powder
- ½ teaspoon coriander

Directions:
1. Combine quinoa, water, kidney beans, diced tomatoes, black beans, corn kernels, olive oil, onion, red bell pepper, garlic cloves, cumin, oregano, chili powder, and coriander in the slow cooker. Mix well.
2. Cover the lid. Cook on low for 8 hours. Best served warm.

Recipe #34 – Slow-Cooked Eggplant

Ingredients:
- 1 cup seitan, thinly sliced
- 1 eggplant, diced
- 1 onion, diced
- ¾ cup split peas
- 2 red chili pepper, sliced
- 2 ½ cups water
- 1 ½ tbsps. molasses
- ½ tsp cumin
- ½ tsp paprika
- 1/8 tsp nutmeg
- 1/8 tsp cinnamon
- Salt
- Mixed herbs
- Freshly ground black pepper, to taste

Directions:
1. Combine all ingredients in a slow cooker. Mix well. Add the mix herb. Season to taste with salt and pepper.
2. Cover and cook on low for 6 hours, stirring once every few hours. Best served warm.

Recipe #35 – Chicken Asparagus

Ingredients:
- 1 pound chicken breasts, sliced into strip
- 2 cloves garlic, chopped finely
- 1 tsp. cornstarch
- 3 tbsps. lemon juice, freshly squeezed
- 1 tsp. lemon zest, grated
- 3 tbsps. soy sauce, reduced-sodium
- 1 carrot, julienned
- 4 scallions, sliced into one-inch diagonal strip
- ¾ pound asparagus, sliced into one-inch diagonal strips

Directions:
1. Combine cornstarch, lemon juice, lemon zest, and soy sauce in a small bowl. Stir in chicken pieces, making sure everything is evenly coated. Cover and place in the refrigerator for 15 minutes.
2. In a slow cooker, stir in garlic, chicken (reserve the marinade), carrots, scallions, and asparagus. Cover the lid. Cook on low for 4 hours.
3. Pour reserved marinade and stir well. Cook for an additional 1 hour.

Recipe #36 – Chicken Mushroom

Ingredients:
- 8 oz cremini mushrooms, sliced
- ¼ tsp. salt
- 1 tsp. mustard, Dijon
- 4 tbsp. flour, all-purpose
- 1 cup chicken broth, reduced-sodium, fat-free
- 1 tsp. cornstarch
- 4 chicken breasts, skinless, boneless
- 2 tsps. canola oil
- ½ cup onion, chopped finely
- ¼ cup sour cream, reduced-fat
- ½ tsp. black pepper, freshly ground

Directions:
1. Place chicken breasts between two plastic wrap sheets and then pound using a meat mallet or rolling pin to flatten them.
2. Combine seasoning and flour in a dish. Dredge flattened chicken breasts on this mixture, making sure to shake off any excess flour.
3. Heat a large skillet (nonstick) on medium-high before pouring in the oil. Once heated, add the chicken and sauté for 3 minutes on each side. Take out from the skillet, then transfer in the slow cooker.

4. Add onion, mushroom, chicken broth, dissolved cornstarch, sour cream and mustard. Cover the lid. Cook on low for 4 hours. Serve with whole grain rice and steamed vegetables.

Recipe #37 – Chickpea Rice

Ingredients:

- 3 cups wild rice, rinsed, drained
- 1 can, 15 oz. chickpea/garbanzos, rinsed, drained
- 1 piece, large carrot, top removed, diced
- 1 piece, large leek, root removed, minced
- 1 Tbsp. cumin powder, add more if desired
- 1 Tbsp. fresh ginger, peeled, grated
- kosher salt
- black pepper, to taste
- Vegetable stock, unsalted
- ¼ cup fresh parsley, minced, divided, for garnish, optional

Directions:

1. Pour ingredients into the slow cooker. Pour stock until liquid reaches 4-cup line of pot. Stir. Cover the lid. Cook on low for 2 hours.
2. Ladle recommended serving portions into bowls. Serve with a sprinkling of fresh parsley on top.

Recipe #38 – Rice Enchilada

Ingredients:

- 2 cups brown short-grained rice, rinsed, drained
- 1 cup frozen sweet corn, thawed, rinsed, drained
- 1 can, 15 oz. cannelloni beans, rinsed, drained
- 1 piece, large green chili, deseeded, minced
- 1 piece, large onion, peeled, minced
- 1½ Tbsp. cumin powder
- ¼ tsp. garlic powder
- Salt, to taste
- Vegetable stock, unsalted
- 1 piece, small lime, sliced into wedges, for serving, optional

Directions:

1. Pour ingredients into the slow cooker. Pour stock until liquid reaches 4-cup line of pot. Stir. Cover the lid. Cook on low for 2 hours.
2. Ladle recommended serving portions into bowls. Serve with lime wedges, if using. Squeeze lime juice over rice before eating.

Recipe #39 – French Beans and Walnuts

Ingredients:

- 2 pieces, large garlic cloves, peeled, minced
- 1 piece, large shallot, peeled, julienned
- 1 piece red chili, deseeded, julienned
- 2 Tbsp. mushroom stock, unsalted
- 1 tsp. fresh ginger, peeled, minced
- ¾ pound French beans, ends and strings removed, rinsed, drained
- ¼ cup garlic roasted walnuts, store-bought, chopped
- Salt
- Mixed herbs
- White pepper, to taste

Directions:

1. Put garlic cloves, ginger, red chili, and shallot. Pour in mushroom stock and add in beans. Cover the lid. Cook on low for 4 hours.
2. Sprinkle in walnuts. Taste and season dish lightly. Divide into equal portions. Serve.

Recipe #40 – Gumbo á La Louisiana

Ingredients:
- 2 tbsp. olive oil
- ¾ cup onion, diced
- 1 tbsp. garlic, minced
- ½ cup green bell pepper, diced
- ½ cup celery, diced
- 6 oz soyrizo
- 5 oz frozen kale
- 5 oz frozen turnip greens
- 5 oz frozen collard greens
- 5 oz frozen spinach
- 2 tbsps. Spelt or whole wheat flour
- 1 jalapeño pepper, seeded, diced
- 3 cups water
- 1 ½ cups green cabbage, shredded
- 2 tbsps. Nutritional yeast
- 2 tbsps. fresh flat parsley, chopped
- ¼ tsp. salt
- 1/8 tsp. freshly ground black pepper

For the Spice and Herb Blend:
- ½ bay leaf
- ¼ tsp. paprika
- 1/8 tsp dried basil
- 1/8 tsp dried thyme
- 1/8 tsp. dried oregano
- 1/8 tsp. cayenne pepper
- 1/8 tsp. garlic powder
- 1/8 tsp. onion powder
- 1/8 tsp. dry mustard

Directions:
1. Chop the greens. Set aside. Combine spice and herb blend. Set aside.
2. Take the soyrizo out of the casings and crumble well. Set aside.
3. Place soyrizo, onion, bell pepper, celery, garlic, jalapeno pepper, water, greens, spice and herb blend, parsley, and nutritional yeast. Cover the lid. Cook on low for 4 hours.
4. Discard bay leaf, then serve right away.

Recipe #41 – Seitan Brisket

Ingredients:
- ½ lb seitan
- 1 carrot, chopped
- ½ celery stalk, diced
- 1 ½ cups vegetable broth
- 1/3 cup red wine
- 1 ½ tbsps. whole wheat flour
- ½ tbsp. soy sauce
- 1 tsp. stevia
- 1 tsp. tomato sauce
- ¼ cup barbecue sauce

Directions:
1. Place celery, carrot, seitan, vegetable broth, red wine, soy sauce, stevia, tomato paste and, flour in a bowl. Mix well.
2. Cover the lid. Cook on low for 4 hours.
3. Add barbecue sauce to the seitan and toss well to combine. Serve seitan with the roasted vegetables.

Recipe #42 – Chili Tofu

Ingredients:
- 28 oz extra firm tofu, drained thoroughly
- 1 tsp. chili garlic paste
- 1 large garlic clove, minced
- 1 ½ tbsp. pure maple syrup
- 1 tbsp. tamari
- 2 tbsps. lime juice, freshly squeezed
- Black pepper
- Coconut oil

Directions:
1. Slice tofu into large cubes and place between two sheets of paper towels. Press gently with a flat plate until most of the water is squeezed out.
2. Combine remaining ingredients in a bowl and season with ground pepper. Then, add the tofu. Turn several times to coat.
3. Cover the bowl with plastic wrap, then refrigerate for at least 4 hours, preferably overnight, to marinate.
4. Once the marinated tofu cubes are ready, place in the slow cooker. Cover the lid and cook on low for 2 hours. Transfer to a serving dish and serve right away.

Recipe #43 – Chickpea Curry

Ingredients:
- 2 onions
- 2 fresh green chilies
- 400g tin chickpeas
- 2 tbsps. sunflower oil
- ½ tsp. asafetida
- 1 tsp. mustard seeds
- 200g tin tomatoes
- 2 tsps. sugar
- 1 tsp. garlic paste
- 1 tsp. fresh ginger paste
- 1 tsp. red chili powder
- 1 tsp. green chili paste
- 1 tsp. dhana jeera powder
- 1 tsp. turmeric
- A few sprigs of coriander
- 2 tsps. sugar
- ½ tsp. garam masala

Directions:
1. Remove skin from the onions and finely slice. Drain chickpeas and rinse. Then, take the green chilies and finely slice.
2. In the slow cooker, add the mustard seeds, asafetida, onions, tomatoes, garlic paste, ginger paste, green chili

paste, dhana jeera, red chili powder, a pinch of sea salt, and sugar. Stir well.
3. Add chickpeas with 250ml of water. Cover the lid and cook on low for 4 hours. To serve, pour the curry into a serving bowl and sprinkle the coriander, garam masala, and green chilies on top.

Recipe# 44 – White Bean and Sweet Potato Chili

Ingredients:
- 2 medium sweet potatoes
- 2 tsps. ground cinnamon
- 1 tbsp. ground cumin
- 1 onion
- 1 tsp. smoked paprika
- 1 fresh red chili
- 1 bunch fresh coriander
- 1 yellow pepper
- 2 red peppers
- 400g tin tomatoes
- 400g tin cannellini beans

Directions:
1. Remove the skin from the sweet potato and chop. Place in the slow cooker. Sprinkle the paprika, cumin, and cinnamon and toss again.
2. Add coriander stalks and leaves, onion, red peppers, yellow pepper, red chili, tomatoes and beans. Add a splash of water.
3. Cover the lid and cook on low for 4 hours. Stir and taste. Adjust seasoning as necessary. Best served over rice and guacamole on the side.

Recipe #45 - Millet with Green Peas and Asparagus

Ingredients:
- ½ cup hulled millet
- 1 cup vegetable broth
- 2 tbsps. lemon juice, freshly squeezed
- 10 asparagus spears, chopped
- ¾ cup frozen green peas
- ¾ tsp. dried thyme
- Sea salt
- Optional: 2 Tbsps. crumbled goat cheese

Directions:
1. Toast the millet in a saucepan for 3 minutes.
2. In the slow cooker, pour broth and add in thyme, freshly squeezed lemon juice, millet, asparagus, and peas. Season with salt and toss to coat.
3. Cover the lid and cook on low for 2 hours.
4. Fold the asparagus and green peas into the millet. Fold in goat cheese, if using, then serve warm.

Recipe #46 – Ginger Broccoli

Ingredients:
- ½ lb frozen broccoli, thawed, chopped
- 1 garlic clove, crushed
- ½ tbsp. fresh ginger, grated
- ½ tbsp. low sodium soy sauce

Directions:
1. Place garlic and chopped broccoli in the slow cooker. Add ginger and soy sauce. Cover the lid and cook on low for 2 hours.
2. Transfer to a serving plate. Serve right away.

Recipe #47 – Soyrizo and Beans

Ingredients:
- ½ tbsp. olive oil
- 6oz soyrizo
- ¾ cup dried red beans, cleaned and rinsed thoroughly
- 2 ¼ cups water
- ¾ cup onion, diced
- 1 tbsp. garlic, minced
- ½ cup green bell pepper, diced
- ½ cup celery, diced
- ½ jalapeno pepper, seeded, minced
- ½ bay leaf
- 1 tsp. dried oregano
- 1/8 tsp. cayenne
- ¼ tsp. salt
- 1/8 tsp. freshly ground black pepper
- Hot pepper sauce

Directions:
1. Remove the soyrizo from the casings and crumble.
2. Place crumbled soyrizo in the slow cooker. Pour in the water, red beans, bell pepper, celery, onion, garlic, jalapeno pepper, bay leaf, chili powder, cayenne, thyme, and oregano.
3. Cover the lid and cook on low for 4 hours.

4. Add hot pepper sauce, salt, and black pepper. Cover the lid and cook for another 1 hour on low. Discard bay leaf. Serve right away.

Recipe #48 – Veggie and Hulled Barley Medley

Ingredients:
- ¾ cup hulled barley
- 2 cups vegetable broth
- ¼ cup carrot, diced
- ¼ cup peas
- ¼ cup green beans, chopped
- ¼ cup corn kernels
- ¼ cup green onion, thinly sliced
- ½ tbsp. nutritional yeast
- ¾ tsp. dill weed
- ½ tsp. garlic powder
- ½ tsp. dried thyme
- Optional: 1 purple kale leaf, chopped
- ½ tsp. salt
- ¼ tsp. freshly ground black pepper

Directions:
1. Rinse barley thoroughly with cold running water in a fine mesh strainer. Drain well and put inside the slow cooker.
2. Add vegetable broth, salt, and pepper to the barley. Mix well. Stir in carrot, green beans, peas, corn, and chopped kale, if using. Add dill weed, nutritional yeast, garlic powder, and thyme. Mix well.

3. Cover the lid and cook on low for 2 hours. Serve right away.

Recipe #49 – Vegetarian Chili

Ingredients:
- 1 tsp. olive oil
- ½ cup TVP granules
- ¾ cup onion, diced
- ½ tbsp. garlic, minced
- 1 ¼ cups water
- 1 tbsp. tomato paste
- ½ tbsp. low sodium soy sauce
- 8 oz tomato sauce
- 2 tsp. cocoa powder
- ½ tbsp. apple cider vinegar

For the Spice Blend:
- ½ tbsp. chili powder
- ½ tsp. cinnamon
- ¼ tsp. paprika
- ¼ tsp. cumin
- 1/8 tsp. cayenne
- ¼ tsp. dried oregano
- 1/8 ts. Cloves allspice
- 1/8 tsp ground cloves
- ½ bay leaf
- ½ tsp. salt
- ¼ tsp ground black pepper

Directions:
1. Pour water, tamari, tomato paste, and TVP in a bowl. Cover and let stand for 10 minutes.
2. Combine the spice blend and set aside.
3. In the meantime, place onions and spice blend into the slow cooker. Add TVP mixture, cocoa powder, tomato sauce, bay leaf, and vinegar. Stir well.
4. Cover the lid and cook on low for 4 hours.
5. Remove bay leaf, then serve, preferably with whole wheat pasta.

Recipe #50 – Stuffed Peppers with Wild Rice and Mushrooms

Ingredients:
- 6 large red bell peppers
- ¾ cup pine nuts
- 1 ½ cups shiitake mushrooms, chopped
- 2 ¼ cups cooked wild rice
- 2/4 cup vegetable broth
- 3 garlic cloves, chopped
- 1/3 tsp. all spice
- 1/3 tsp. turmeric
- 1 tsp. salt

Directions:
1. Put garlic, mushrooms, pine nuts, spices, and salt in a saucepan. Sauté until the pine nuts become lightly toasted.
2. Transfer in the slow cooker. Add broth, cooked wild rice, and bell peppers.
3. Cover the lid and cook on low for 4 hours. Arrange in the prepared dish. Serve.

Chapter 3 – Delicious Homemade Slow Cooker Condiments

Fruit Jam Recipes

These make multiple servings; recommended serving size is 1½ to 2 tablespoons per serving. Spread on multigrain bread.

Recipe #51 - Balsamic Apricot Jam

Ingredients:

- 3 Tbsps. balsamic vinegar
- 2 pounds apricots, unpeeled, pitted, diced
- 1 cup raw organic honey
- ¼ cup water
- ½ piece large lemon, fresh juiced, pips removed

Directions:

1. Place ingredients in the slow cooker.
2. Roughly mash fruits using a wooden spoon. Cover the lid and cook on low for 2 hours.
3. Cool to room temperature before storing in airtight container; use as needed.

Recipe #52 – Balsamic Blackberry Jam

Ingredients:

- 3 Tbsps. balsamic vinegar, preferably aged
- 2½ pounds frozen blackberries, thawed
- 1 cup raw organic honey
- ¼ cup water
- ½ piece large lemon, fresh juiced, pips removed

Directions:

1. Place ingredients in the slow cooker.
2. Using potato masher, mash berries. Cover the lid and cook on low for 2 hours.
3. Cool to room temperature before storing in airtight container; use as needed.

Recipe #53 – Balsamic Cranberry Jam

Ingredients:

- 3 Tbsps. balsamic vinegar
- 2½ pounds frozen cranberries, thawed
- 1 cup raw organic honey
- ¼ cup water
- ½ piece large lemon, fresh juiced, pips removed

Directions:

1. Place ingredients in the slow cooker.
2. Using potato masher, mash berries. Cover the lid and cook on low for 2 hours.
3. Cool to room temperature before storing in airtight container; use as needed.

Recipe #54 – 21 Balsamic Strawberry Jam

Ingredients:

- 3 Tbsps. balsamic vinegar
- 2½ pounds frozen strawberries, thawed
- 1 cup raw organic honey
- ¼ cup water
- ½ piece large lemon, fresh juiced, pips removed

Directions:

1. Place ingredients in the slow cooker.
2. Using potato masher, mash berries. Cover the lid and cook on low for 2 hours.
3. Cool to room temperature before storing in airtight container; use as needed.

Recipe #55 – Blueberry and Raspberry Jam

Ingredients:

- 3 cups frozen blueberries, thawed
- 3 cups frozen raspberries, thawed
- 1 cup raw organic honey
- ¼ cup water
- 1 Tbsp. lemon juice, fresh squeezed

Directions:

1. Place ingredients in the slow cooker.
2. Using potato masher, mash berries. Cover the lid and cook on low for 2 hours.
3. Cool to room temperature before storing in airtight container; use as needed.

Recipe #56 – Blackberry and Strawberry Jam

Ingredients:

- 3 cups frozen blueberries, thawed
- 1 cup raw organic honey
- ¼ cup water
- ½ pound froze strawberries, thawed
- 1 Tbsp. lemon juice, fresh squeezed, pips removed

Directions:

1. Place ingredients in the slow cooker.
2. Using potato masher, mash berries. Cover the lid and cook on low for 2 hours.
3. Cool to room temperature before storing in airtight container; use as needed.

Recipe #57 – Chia Seeds Blueberry Jam

Ingredients:

- 3 cups fresh blueberries
- 1 cup raw organic honey
- ¼ cup water
- 2 Tbsps. chia seeds
- 1 Tbsp. lemon juice, fresh squeezed

Directions:

1. Place ingredients in the slow cooker.
2. Using potato masher, mash berries. Cover the lid and cook on low for 2 hours.
3. Cool to room temperature before storing in airtight container; use as needed.

Recipe #58 – Apricot Jam

Ingredients:

- 2 pounds apricots, unpeeled, pitted, diced
- 1 cup raw organic honey
- ¼ cup water
- ½ piece, large lemon, fresh juiced, pips removed
- Pinch of salt

Directions:

1. Place ingredients in the slow cooker.
2. Using potato masher, mash berries. Cover the lid and cook on low for 2 hours.
3. Cool to room temperature before storing in airtight container; use as needed.

Recipe #59 – Cinnamon Apricot Jam

Ingredients:

- 2 pounds apricots, unpeeled, pitted, diced
- 2 Tbsps. cinnamon powder
- 1 cup raw organic honey
- ¼ cup water
- ½ piece large lemon, fresh juiced, pips removed
- Pinch of salt

Directions:

1. Place ingredients in the slow cooker.
2. Using potato masher, mash berries. Cover the lid and cook on low for 2 hours.
3. Cool to room temperature before storing in airtight container; use as needed.

Recipe #60 – Blueberry Jam

Ingredients:

- 2½ pounds frozen blueberries, thawed
- 1 cup raw organic honey
- ¼ cup water
- ½ piece large lemon, fresh juiced, pips removed
- Pinch of salt

Directions:

1. Place ingredients in the slow cooker.
2. Using potato masher, mash berries. Cover the lid and cook on low for 2 hours.
3. Cool to room temperature before storing in airtight container; use as needed.

Recipe #61 – Easy Mango Jam

Ingredients:

- 4 pieces large ripe mangoes, peeled, pitted, flesh diced
- 1 piece small lime, fresh squeezed, pips removed
- ¾ cup honey
- ¼ cup water
- Pinch of salt

Directions:

1. Place ingredients in the slow cooker.
2. Using potato masher, mash berries. Cover the lid and cook on low for 2 hours.
3. Cool to room temperature before storing in airtight container; use as needed.

Recipe #62 – Cinnamon Cranberry Jam

Ingredients:

- 2½ pound fresh cranberries, rinsed well, drained
- 2 tsps. cinnamon powder
- 1 cup raw organic honey
- ¼ cup water
- ½ piece large lemon, fresh juiced, pips removed
- Pinch of salt

Directions:

1. Place ingredients in the slow cooker.
2. Using potato masher, mash berries. Cover the lid and cook on low for 2 hours.
3. Cool to room temperature before storing in airtight container; use as needed.

Recipe #63 – Blackberry Jam

Ingredients:

- 2½ pounds frozen blackberries, thawed
- 1 cup raw organic honey
- ¼ cup water
- ½ piece large lemon, fresh juiced, pips removed
- Pinch of sea salt

Directions:

1. Place ingredients in the slow cooker.
2. Using potato masher, mash berries. Cover the lid and cook on low for 2 hours.
3. Cool to room temperature before storing in airtight container; use as needed.

Recipe #64 – Cherry Jam

Ingredients:

- 2 pounds cherries, stemmed, pitted, halved
- 1 cup raw organic honey
- ¼ cup water
- ½ piece large lemon, fresh juiced, pips removed
- Pinch of sea salt

Directions:

1. Place ingredients in the slow cooker.
2. Using potato masher, mash berries. Cover the lid and cook on low for 2 hours.
3. Cool to room temperature before storing in airtight container; use as needed.

Recipe #65 – Pineapple Jam

Ingredients:

- 3 pieces large lime, fresh squeezed, pips removed
- 1 piece small fresh, slightly overripe pineapple, peeled, eyes removed, cored, pulp diced
- 1 cup raw organic honey
- ¼ cup water
- Pinch of sea salt

Directions:

1. Place ingredients in the slow cooker.
2. Using potato masher, mash berries. Cover the lid and cook on low for 2 hours.
3. Cool to room temperature before storing in airtight container; use as needed.

Recipe #66 – Peach Jam

Ingredients:

- 2 pounds peaches, unpeeled, pitted, cubed
- 1 cup raw organic honey
- ¼ cup water
- ½ piece large lemon, fresh juiced, pips removed
- Pinch of sea salt

Directions:

1. Place ingredients in the slow cooker.
2. Using potato masher, mash berries. Cover the lid and cook on low for 2 hours.
3. Cool to room temperature before storing in airtight container; use as needed.

Recipe #67 – Raspberry Jam

Ingredients:

- 2½ pounds frozen raspberries, thawed
- 1 cup raw organic honey
- ¼ cup water
- ½ piece large lemon, fresh juiced, pips removed
- Pinch of salt

Directions:

1. Place ingredients in the slow cooker.
2. Using potato masher, mash berries. Cover the lid and cook on low for 2 hours.
3. Cool to room temperature before storing in airtight container; use as needed.

Recipe #68 – Plum Jam

Ingredients:

- 2 pounds plums, unpeeled, pitted, diced
- 1 cup raw organic honey
- ¼ cup water
- ½ piece large lemon, fresh juiced, pips removed
- Pinch of salt

Directions:

1. Place ingredients in the slow cooker.
2. Using potato masher, mash berries. Cover the lid and cook on low for 2 hours.
3. Cool to room temperature before storing in airtight container; use as needed.

Recipe #69 – Berry Jam

Ingredients:

- 1 piece small lemon, fresh juiced, pips removed
- 1 cup frozen gooseberries, thawed
- 1 cup frozen blackberries, thawed
- 1 cup frozen dewberries, thawed
- 1 cup frozen blueberries, thawed
- 1 cup frozen boysenberries, thawed
- 1 cup frozen loganberries, thawed
- 1 cup water
- 1 cup honey
- Pinch of salt

Directions:

1. Place ingredients in the slow cooker.
2. Using potato masher, mash berries. Cover the lid and cook on low for 2 hours.
3. Cool to room temperature before storing in airtight container; use as needed.

Recipe #70 – Strawberry Jam

Ingredients:

- 2½ pounds frozen strawberries, thawed, quartered
- 1 cup raw organic honey
- ¼ cup water
- ½ piece large lemon, fresh juiced, pips removed
- Pinch of salt

Directions:

1. Place ingredients in the slow cooker.
2. Using potato masher, mash berries. Cover the lid and cook on low for 2 hours.
3. Cool to room temperature before storing in airtight container; use as needed.

Recipe #71 – Basil-Pumpkin Pesto Sauce

Ingredients:

- 5 pieces large garlic cloves, peeled, minced
- 2 Tbsps. lemon juice, freshly squeezed
- 1 cup packed basil leaves, rinsed, spun-dried
- ²/₃ cup extra virgin olive oil
- ¼ cup toasted pumpkin seeds, shelled, store-bough
- kosher salt
- white pepper, to taste

Directions:

1. Place ingredients into the slow cooker. Cover the lid and cook on low for 2 hours.
2. Allow to cool and then put inside a food processor. Process until smooth. Season lightly. Drizzle lightly on toast

Recipe #72 – Basil-Walnut Pesto Sauce

Ingredients:

- 5 pieces large garlic cloves, peeled, minced
- 2 Tbsps. lemon juice, freshly squeezed
- 1 cup packed basil leaves, rinsed, spun-dried
- 2/3 cup extra virgin olive oil
- 1/3 cup walnuts, shelled, toasted well on dry pan
- Salt
- white pepper, to taste

Directions:

1. Place ingredients in the slow cooker.
2. Using potato masher, mash berries. Cover the lid and cook on low for 2 hours.
3. Cool to room temperature before storing in airtight container; use as needed.

Recipe #73 – Tomato Pesto Sauce

Ingredients:

- 5 pieces, large garlic cloves, peeled, minced
- 2 Tbsps. lemon juice, freshly squeezed
- 2/3 cup, loosely packed basil leaves, rinsed, spun-dried
- 2/3 cup extra virgin olive oil
- 1/3 cup pine nuts, toasted well on dry pan
- 1/3 cup sun-dried tomatoes, store-bought, chopped
- Salt
- white pepper, to taste

Directions:

1. Place ingredients in the slow cooker.
2. Using potato masher, mash berries. Cover the lid and cook on low for 2 hours.
3. Cool to room temperature before storing in airtight container; use as needed.

Recipe #74 – Cilantro Pesto Sauce

Ingredients:

- 5 pieces large garlic cloves, peeled, minced
- 2 Tbsps. lemon juice, freshly squeezed
- 1 cup packed cilantro leaves, rinsed, spun-dried
- ⅔ cup extra virgin olive oil
- ⅓ cup pine nuts, toasted well on dry pa
- Salt
- white pepper, to taste

Directions:

1. Place ingredients in the slow cooker.
2. Using potato masher, mash berries. Cover the lid and cook on low for 2 hours.
3. Cool to room temperature before storing in airtight container; use as needed.

Recipe #75 – Cilantro-Cashew Pesto Sauce

Ingredients:

- 5 pieces large garlic cloves, peeled, minced
- 2 Tbsps. lemon juice, freshly squeezed
- 1 cup packed cilantro leaves, rinsed, spun-dried
- 2/3 cup extra virgin olive oil
- 1/3 cup cashew nuts, shelled, toasted well on dry pa
- Salt
- white pepper, to taste

Directions:

1. Place ingredients in the slow cooker.
2. Using potato masher, mash berries. Cover the lid and cook on low for 2 hours.
3. Cool to room temperature before storing in airtight container; use as needed.

Recipe #76 – Cilantro-Walnut Pesto Sauce

Ingredients:

- 5 pieces large garlic cloves, peeled, minced
- 2 Tbsps. lemon juice, freshly squeezed
- 1 cup packed cilantro leaves, rinsed, spun-dried
- $2/3$ cup extra virgin olive oil
- $1/3$ cup walnuts, shelled, toasted well on dry pan
- Salt
- white pepper, to taste

Directions:

1. Place ingredients in the slow cooker.
2. Using potato masher, mash berries. Cover the lid and cook on low for 2 hours.
3. Cool to room temperature before storing in airtight container; use as needed.

Recipe #77 – Kale Pesto Sauce

Ingredients:

- 5 pieces large garlic cloves, peeled, minced
- 2 Tbsps. lemon juice, freshly squeezed
- 1 cup packed basil leaves, rinsed, spun-dried
- ½ cup packed kale leaves, tough stems removed, torn, rinsed, spun-dried
- ¾ cup extra virgin olive oil
- ⅓ cup pine nuts, toasted well on dry pan
- Salt
- white pepper, to taste

Directions:

1. Place ingredients in the slow cooker.
2. Using potato masher, mash berries. Cover the lid and cook on low for 2 hours.
3. Cool to room temperature before storing in airtight container; use as needed.

Recipe #78 – Kale-Cashew Pesto Sauce

Ingredients:

- 5 pieces large garlic cloves, peeled, minced
- 2 Tbsps. lemon juice, freshly squeezed
- 1 cup packed basil leaves, rinsed, spun-dried
- ½ cup packed kale leaves, tough stems removed, torn, rinsed, spun-dried
- ¾ cup extra virgin olive oil
- ⅓ cup cashew nuts, toasted well on dry pan
- Salt
- white pepper, to taste

Directions:

1. Place ingredients in the slow cooker.
2. Using potato masher, mash berries. Cover the lid and cook on low for 2 hours.
3. Cool to room temperature before storing in airtight container; use as needed.

Recipe #79 – Kale-Walnut Pesto Sauce

Ingredients:

- 5 pieces large garlic cloves, peeled, minced
- 2 Tbsps. lemon juice, freshly squeezed
- ½ cup packed kale leaves, tough stems removed, torn, rinsed, spun-dried
- ¾ cup extra virgin olive oil
- 1/3 cup walnuts, shelled, toasted well on dry pan
- Salt
- white pepper, to taste

Directions:

1. Place ingredients in the slow cooker.
2. Using potato masher, mash berries. Cover the lid and cook on low for 2 hours.
3. Cool to room temperature before storing in airtight container; use as needed.

Recipe #80 – Mint Pesto Sauce

Ingredients:

- 5 pieces large garlic cloves, peeled, minced
- 2 Tbsps. lemon juice, freshly squeezed
- 1 cup packed mint leaves, rinsed, spun-dried
- 2/3 cup extra virgin olive oil
- 1/3 cup pine nuts, toasted well on dry pa
- Salt
- white pepper, to taste

Directions:

1. Place ingredients in the slow cooker.
2. Using potato masher, mash berries. Cover the lid and cook on low for 2 hours.
3. Cool to room temperature before storing in airtight container; use as needed.

Chapter 4 – Crockpot Dinner Selections

Recipe #81 – Coconut and Ginger Linguine

Ingredients
- 8 oz dry linguine
- 1 cup spinach leaves, rinsed and drained
- ½ cup Swiss chard, rinsed and dried
- ½ tbsp. olive oil
- 2 small garlic cloves, minced
- 1 ½ tbsps. fresh ginger, grated
- 8 oz coconut milk
- ¼ tsp. stevia
- 1 ½ tsps. lemon juice, freshly squeezed
- Red pepper flakes
- Salt
- Mixed herbs
- Ground black pepper

Directions:
1. Cook the pasta based on the package instructions. Rinse over cold water, drain thoroughly, and set aside.
2. Meanwhile, place garlic, ginger, stevia, coconut milk, in the slow cooker. Mix well. Season with red pepper flakes, salt, mixed herbs. and pepper. Add spinach and Swiss chard. Cover the lid. Cook on low for 4 hours.

3. Let it cool, then pour into a blender or food processor. Blend until creamy.
4. Transfer the pasta into a serving bowl, then add the sauce. Toss well to coat, then serve right away with grated parmesan.

Recipe #82 – Vegan Mac 'n' Cheese

Ingredients:
- 6 oz whole wheat rotini
- 2 ½ tbsps. nutritional yeast
- 2 ½ tbsps. non0dairy butter
- ½ panko breadcrumbs
- 1 cup broccoli, chopped, steamed
- ½ cup sweet potato, diced
- ½ carrot, diced
- ½ cup water
- ½ tbsp. miso paste
- ½ tbsp. lemon juice, freshly squeezed
- ½ tbsp. tahini
- ½ tsp. Dijon mustard
- 2 tbsps. cashews, chopped
- ½ tsp. salt

Directions:
1. Cook the pasta based on the package instructions. Rinse over cold water, drain thoroughly, and set aside.
2. In a slow cooker, combine carrot and sweet potato. Add the remaining ingredients, except for breadcrumbs and pasta. Cover the lid. Cook on low for 4 hours.
3. Allow to cool and then transfer in a food processor. Blend until smooth.
4. Transfer in a casserole dish. Top with the panko breadcrumbs. Bake for 15 minutes, or until top is golden brown. Best served warm.

Recipe #83 – Barley and Butternut Squash Casserole

Ingredients:
- 1 tbsp. olive oil
- 1tbsp. non-dairy butter
- ½ cup pearl barley
- 1 ¾ cups butternut squash, cubed
- 1 garlic clove, minced
- ½ red onion, minced
- 1 tbsp. whole wheat flour
- 1 cup nonodairy milk
- 1 tsp. dried rosemary
- ½ cup non-dairy cheddar cheese, shredded
- 1/3 cup Parmesan cheese, shredded
- Nutmeg
- ¼ tsp. sea salt
- Ground black pepper

Directions:
1. Combine water and barley in the slow cooker. Add garlic, onion, squash, butter, flour, milk, rosemary, and a dash of nutmeg in the slow cooker. Season to taste with salt and pepper.
2. Cover the lid and cook on low for 2 hours.
3. Mix together the squash, barley and sauce in a baking dish, then top with Parmesan cheese. Seal with aluminum foil and bake for 15 minutes.

4. Uncover and set the oven to broil. Broil for 3 minutes, or until the casserole is golden brown. Let cool for 10 minutes, then serve.

Recipe #84 – Seitan in Soy Yogurt

Ingredients:
- ½ lb. seitan
- 1 onion, diced
- 2 garlic cloves
- 2 ½ tbsps. soy yogurt
- 2 ½ tbsps. tomato sauce
- ½ tsp. cumin
- ¼ tsp. cayenne pepper
- 1 fresh clove
- ½ tsp. salt

Directions:
1. Slice seitan into bite-sized cubes and set aside.
1. If using wooden skewers, soak them in cold water.
2. Combine yogurt, tomato sauce, onion, garlic, cumin, cayenne, and clove in the slow cooker. Cover the lid and cook on low for 2 hours.
3. Allow to cool and then pour in a food processor. Blend until smooth.
4. Transfer mixture into a bowl, then place the seitan in it. Turn to coat. Best served warm.

Recipe #85 – Yummy Glazed Salmon

Ingredients:
- ¼ cup soy sauce, reduced-sodium
- 1 tbsp. lime juice
- 2 tbsps. syrup, ample
- 2 tbsps. scallions, chopped
- 4 fillets, salmon
- 1 tbsp. ginger, freshly grated

Directions:
1. Mix soy sauce, maple syrup, and lime juice in a mixing bowl. Add scallions and ginger, stirring well to combine. Stir in the salmon fillets and coat well with the mixture.
2. Transfer in the slow cooker. Cover the lid and cook on low for 6 hours. Best served warm.

Recipe #86 – Cranberry-Apple Pork

Ingredients:
- 2 apples, Granny Smith, peeled, cored, sliced thickly
- 1 tablespoon sugar, brown
- 1 cup cranberries, fresh
- 2 pork tenderloins, one-pounder, w/ sliver skin and fat trimmed
- ½ cup cider
- 2 tablespoons cider vinegar
- 1 teaspoon cinnamon

Directions:
1. Place tenderloins inside the slow cooker. Arrange apple slices around the pork. Scatter cranberries.
2. Pour in cider vinegar and apple cider, then dust the surface of the pork with cinnamon and sugar.
3. Cover the lid and cook on low for 8 hours. Let stand for ten minutes. Serve.

Recipe #87 – Herbed Tenderloin

Ingredients:

- ¼ cup mixed herbs (thyme, parsley, rosemary, sage), fresh, chopped finely
- ¾ cup pork tenderloin
- ½ teaspoon black pepper, freshly ground

Directions:

1. Coat pork with the herbs. Tuck in thin ends to make sure the pork evenly cooks.
2. Place pork in the slow cooker. Cover the lid and cook on low for 8 hours or on high for 4 hours.
3. Let stand for ten minutes. Serve.

Recipe #88 – Guilt-Free Stroganoff

Ingredients:
- 8 oz mushrooms, cremini, sliced
- ½ cup shallots, chopped
- 1 tablespoon cornstarch, mixed w/ ¼ cup water
- ¾ pound steak, top round, w/ fat trimmed
- 1 ¼ cups beef broth, low-sodium, fat-free
- 1 tablespoon mustard, Dijon
- 4 servings noodles, wide, cooked (8 oz uncooked)
- ½ cup yogurt, plain, low-fat (mixed w/ ½ teaspoon cornstarch)

Directions:
1. Slice beef into extremely thin slices, cut into bite-sized pieces. Transfer in the slow cooker.
2. Add in mushrooms, shallots, broth, mustard, cornstarch, and yogurt. Stir well. Cover the lid and cook on low for 2 hours.
3. Serve over hot noodles.

Recipe #89 – Slow-Cooked Rice and Bean Dish

Ingredients:

- 3 cups white long-grained Japanese sticky rice, rinsed, drained
- 1 can, 15 oz. black beans, unseasoned, rinsed, drained
- 1 Tbsp., heaping garlic-roasted cashew nuts, store-bought, roughly chopped
- ⅛ tsp. cumin powder
- ⅛ tsp. onion powder
- ⅛ tsp. Spanish paprika powder
- Salt
- Black pepper, to taste
- Mushroom stock

Directions:

1. Pour ingredients into the slow cooker. Pour stock until liquid reaches 4-cup line of pot. Stir.
2. Cover the lid and cook on low for 4 hours.
3. Ladle recommended serving portions into bowls. Serve warm.

Recipe #90 – Corn and Mushroom

Ingredients:

- 2 Tbsps. vegetable stock, unsalted
- 1 Tbsp. coconut oil, organic
- 2 cans, 15 oz. each whole corn kernels, rinsed, drained
- 1 can, 15 oz. button mushrooms, pieces and stems, rinsed, drained
- 1 piece, large shallot, peeled, mince
- Salt
- White pepper, to taste

Directions:

1. Pour ingredients into the slow cooker. Pour stock until liquid reaches 4-cup line of pot. Stir.
2. Cover the lid and cook on low for 4 hours.
3. Divide into equal portions. Serve

Recipe #91 – Three Bean Chili

Ingredients:
- 15 oz black beans, reduced, drained, rinsed
- ¾ pound beef, ground, extra-lean
- 15 oz pinto beans, reduced-sodium, drained, rinsed
- 2 carrots, diced
- 4 oz jalapeno peppers, diced, drained
- 1 tbsp. chili powder
- 1 onion, chopped
- 2 tsps. cumin powder
- 15 oz kidney beans, reduced-sodium, drained, rinsed
- 28 oz tomatoes, crushed

Directions:
1. Add carrots, onions, ground beef, cumin, chili powder, black beans, kidney beans, pinto beans, crushed tomatoes, and jalapeno peppers in the slow cooker.
2. Cover the lid and cook on low for 8 hours. Serve.

Recipe #92 – Butternut Squash and Beef Stew

Ingredients:
- 4 oz carrots, sliced into chunks
- 1 onion, large, sliced
- 2 tsps. Worcestershire sauce
- 1 butternut squash
- 1 tsp. dried thyme
- ¾ lb stewing beef, lean, w/ excess fat trimmed
- 8 oz cremini mushrooms, sliced
- 14 oz tomatoes, crushed
- 1 tsp. dried oregano

Directions:

1. Add all ingredients in the slow cooker. Cover the lid and cook on low for 8 hours or on high for 4 hours. Serve right away.

Recipe #93 – Sweet Corn-Bean-Beef Chili

Ingredients:
- ½ pound beef, ground, extra-lean
- 1 green pepper, small, chopped
- 2 tsp. cumin
- 15 oz pinto beans
- 1 Serrano chile/jalapeno, chopped finely
- 1 onion, medium, chopped finely
- 1 tbsp. chili powder
- 15 oz tomatoes, crushed
- 1 ½ cups sweet corn, frozen

Directions:
1. Combine all ingredients in the slow cooker.
2. Cover the lid and cook on low for 8 hours. Serve immediately.

Recipe #94 – Veggie Curry

Ingredients:
- 1 cup beans, green, trimmed, sliced into two-inch cuts
- 1 tbsp. cumin
- 2 carrots, sliced
- 1 cup cauliflower/broccoli florets
- 2 tbsps. curry powder
- 14 ½ oz tomatoes, diced, w/out added salt
- 1 onion, chopped
- 1 potato, cubed
- 1 butternut squash, cubed
- 8 oz tomato sauce, w/out added salt

Directions:
1. In a slow cooker, stir in cumin, curry powder, potatoes, carrots, onion, broccoli, green beans, squash, tomato sauce, tomatoes, and the rest of the vegetables.
2. Cover the lid and cook on low for 2 hours. Once the sauce has thickened and the vegetables have tenderized, pour onto cooked whole grain rice and serve.

Recipe #95 – Tasty Farfelle

Ingredients:
- ¼ cup Parmesan cheese, freshly grated
- 1 lb, asparagus spears, sliced into 1 ½-inch cuts
- ¼ cup fresh basil, chopped finely
- ¼ cup shallots, minced
- 12 ounces, whole wheat farfelle pasta
- 2 cloves garlic, crushed
- 1 pint cherry tomatoes, halved
- 2 tbsps. balsamic vinegar
- ½ tsp. freshly ground black pepper

Directions:
1. Except for the pasta, pour all ingredients in the slow cooker. Cover the lid and cook on low for 4 hours.
2. Meanwhile, follow package directions in cooking the pasta. Drain cooked pasta, then place in a pasta bowl along with a little liquid.
3. After 4 hours, pour sauce onto the pasta mixture. Sprinkle with cheese and serve right away.

Recipe #96 – Scrumptious Lentil Soup

Ingredients:
- 1 cup onion
- 1 cup carrots, diced
- ¾ cup celery, chopped
- 15 oz tomatoes, crushed
- 1 cup brown/green lentils, rinsed
- 1 tbsp. curry powder
- 3 cups vegetable broth, low-sodium, fat-free

Directions:
1. In the slow cooker, stir in onions, carrots, and celery, tomatoes, lentils, and curry powder. Pour in the broth.
2. Cover the lid and cook on low for 2 hours. Serve right away.

Recipe #97 – Pumpkin Soup

Ingredients:
- 2 cloves garlic, minced
- 1 yellow onion, finely chopped
- 1 tsp. cumin
- 1 tbsp. curry powder
- 15 oz pumpkin
- 3 cups vegetable/chicken broth, low-sodium, fat-free
- 12 oz milk, fat-free, evaporated
- ½ tsp. black pepper, freshly ground

Directions:
1. In a slow cooker, stir in garlic, onion, cumin, curry powder, pumpkin, chicken broth, milk, and pepper.
2. Cover the lid and cook on low for 2 hours.
3. Allow to cool and then transfer in a blender. Process until smooth. Serve.

Recipe #98 – Savory Roasted Cabbage

Ingredients:
- ¼ green cabbage head
- ¼ red cabbage head
- 1 tbsp. olive oil
- 1 tbsp. balsamic vinegar
- Salt
- Ground black pepper

Directions:
1. Chop the cabbages and arrange in the slow cooker. Drizzle olive oil on top and toss well to coat. Season with salt and pepper, then toss again.
2. Cover the lid and cook on low for 2 hours.
3. Remove from the slow cooker and drizzle the balsamic vinegar on top. Toss well, then serve right away.

Recipe #99 – Thai Tofu Bowls

Ingredients:
- ½ tsp olive oil
- 24 oz extra firm tofu, cubed
- 1 ½ cups vegetable broth
- 1 cup cauliflower, chopped
- 3 tbsps. scallions, chopped
- 1 garlic clove, crushed
- ¼ cup onion, chopped
- 1 tsp. ginger grated
- 1 celery stalk, sliced
- ½ tbsp. lemon juice, freshly squeezed
- ½ tsp. five spice
- 1/ tsp hot pepper sauce
- ¼ tsp salt
- 3 tbsps. fresh cilantro, chopped

Directions:
1. Place tofu cubes in the slow cooker. Add onion, garlic, celery, lemon juice, salt, ginger, and five spice. Mix well.
2. Stir hot pepper sauce in the broth until thoroughly combined, then pour into the slow cooker. Shred cauliflower in the food processor until grainy. Put inside the slow cooker.
3. Cover the lid and cook on low for 4 hours.

4. Divide mixture among bowls. Garnish with cilantro. Serve.

Recipe #100 – Sweet Potato and Beef

Ingredients:
- 8 oz button mushrooms, halved
- 1 cup red wine
- 1 onion, roughly chopped
- 2 bay leaves
- 2 celery stalks, sliced
- 1 tsp. dried thyme
- 2 cups sweet potato, chopped
- 2 tbsps. tomato paste
- 1 garlic clove, crushed
- 8 oz tomato sauce, w/out added salt
- 2/3 lb stewing beef, lean
- 2 carrots, sliced
- 15 oz black beans, reduced-sodium, drained, rinsed
- 1 tsp. dried oregano

Directions:
1. Fill the slow cooker with vegetables before adding in the beef. Pour red wine, bay leaves, black beans, tomato sauce, tomato paste, and herbs.
2. Cover the lid. Allow the mixture to cook for eight hours on low. Serve.

Conclusion

Thank you again for buying the book.

I hope this book was able to help you expand your culinary repertoire when it comes to crockpot dishes. Cooking effortlessly has never been this good! Not only will you be eating healthy and flavorful meals, but you also eliminate wasting precious hours preparing a meal.

The next step is to try these crockpot recipes if you haven't already and be amazed how this simple kitchen appliance can dish up amazing food.

If you found this book enjoyable and useful, I would be grateful if you could please take a few minutes to post a review on Amazon and share your thoughts with me and other readers.

Many thanks for your support and I wish you a healthy, loving, peaceful, and happy life!

Part 2

BEEF RECIPES

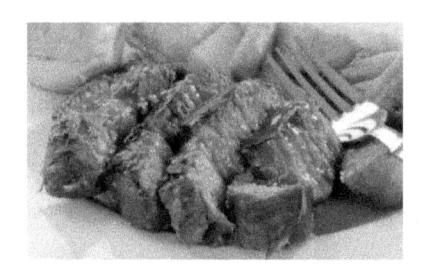

Crock Pot Beef Stew

Who doesn't love beef stew? It is hearty and the meat just melts away in your mouth. This easy recipe will provide your whole family with a delicious Sunday dinner.

Ingredients:
2 pounds beef chuck, chopped into 1 inch cubes
1/3 cup flour
1 tablespoon olive oil
1/2 teaspoon pepper
1/2 teaspoon seasoned salt
2 teaspoons smoked paprika (if unavailable, use regular paprika)
1 (8 ounce) package mushrooms, diced
1 large onion, chopped
2 garlic cloves, minced
5 carrots, peeled and sliced
2 potatoes, peeled and chopped

2 celery stalk, diced
1 tablespoon Worcestershire sauce
1/4 cup Marsala wine
1 (14 1/2 ounce) can crushed tomatoes
3 (10 1/2 ounce) cans beef broth, low sodium
1 (1 ounce) package onion soup mix, dried

Optional Ingredients:
Additional salt and pepper, to taste
2 tablespoons water
2 tablespoons cornstarch

Directions:

In a large bag, combine the seasoned salt, flour, pepper, and 1 teaspoon paprika. Add in the beef chunks and shake to coat all pieces.

Grab a large skillet and allow the oil to heat over medium high heat. Once hot, add in the beef shaking off any excess flour. Stir in the mushrooms and onion. Cook until the beef is evenly browned on all sides and is no longer pink. Drain and then place the beef mixture into your crock pot.

Add in the wine, potatoes, celery, carrots, Worcestershire sauce, and garlic. Stir well. Pour the beef broth and tomatoes over top of the mixture and stir well. Add in the remaining paprika and onion soup mix. Stir. Cover and cook on HIGH for 4-6 hours. (You can also cook on LOW for 10-12 hours.) Season as needed with salt and pepper.

(If you want a thick stew, mix together the water and cornstarch in a small bowl until blended. During the last five minutes of cooking, slowly stir into the stew until thickened.)

If you are short on time and don't mind if your meat doesn't have the seared brown look, you can skip browning the beef in the skillet. Omit the flour and place the roast in the slow cooker. Follow the rest of the instructions to cook.

Nutritional Information per Serving:
Servings: 6
Calories: 467
Fat: 20.6g
Carbohydrates: 43.8g
Protein: 25.3g

Beef Stew Shopping List:
Beef chuck roast (2 pounds)
Mushrooms (8 ounces)
Garlic cloves
Carrots (5)
Potatoes (2)
Celery
Marsala wine

Staples/Seasonings:
Flour
Olive oil
Pepper
Salt
Smoked (or regular) paprika

Worcestershire sauce
Crushed tomatoes, 14 ½ ounce can
Low sodium beef broth 3 (10 ½ ounce) cans
Onion soup mix

Our Go-To Recipe for Shredded Beef

This recipe is one of the best for delicious shredded beef. You can enjoy the scents as it fills your home throughout the day. Serve the beef on bread and you have the perfect meal. If you have any leftovers, this is a great recipe to use for *Mouthwatering Beef Nachos.*

Ingredients:
1 (3-4 pound) round roast, boneless
2 tablespoons Worcestershire sauce
1 tablespoon Montreal steak seasoning
1 cup beef broth, low sodium

Directions:
Lay the roast into your slow cooker and pour the beef broth over top of it. Add in the Worcestershire sauce and steak seasoning. Cover. Cook on HIGH for 4 hours. (You can also cook it on HIGH for 6 to 8 hours)

Shred the beef with two forks toward the end of the cooking time. Finish cooking and serve.

Nutritional Information per Serving:

Servings: 6-8
Calories: 100
Fat: 3g
Carbohydrates: 1g
Protein: 13g

Shredded Beef Recipe Shopping List:
1 (3-4 pound) round roast, boneless

Staples/Seasonings (if you don't have, you'll need these also):
Worcestershire sauce
Montreal steak seasoning
Low sodium beef broth

Slow Cooked Shredded Spicy Beef

This shredded beef makes a great sandwich for lunch. Top it with some cabbage and shredded carrots for a complete meal.

Ingredients:
2 ½ pounds beef chuck, bone-in
7 ounces salsa, hot
1 (14.5 ounce) can diced tomatoes
1 large onion, chopped
1 (4 ounce) can diced green chilies, drained
3 garlic cloves, minced
2 cups beef broth, low sodium
1 tablespoon honey

1 teaspoon ground cumin
2 ½ teaspoons salt
2 tablespoons chili powder

Directions:
Grab the beef and then rinse it off under cool water. Pat it dry and trim off any extra fat that is present. Place the beef in your slow cooker. Add in the salsa, tomatoes, onion, chilies, chili powder, garlic, salt, honey, and cumin. Slowly pour the beef broth over top of all of the ingredients.

Cover your slow cooker and cook on LOW for 8 to 10 hours. (If you want a thick sauce, remove the lid during the last 30 minutes of cook time.) Remove the beef from the slow cooker and place on a carving dish. Shred the meat and discard the bone.

If desired, use a large spoon and reserve half of the sauce from the slow cooker to use on top of rice or as a dipping sauce for the sandwiches.

Return the beef to the slow cooker and stir to coat with the sauce. Cover and allow to warm.

Then serve on sandwich buns.

Nutritional Information per Serving:
Servings: 6-8
Calories: 261
Fat: 11g
Carbohydrates: 10g
Protein: 30g

Spicy Shredded Beef Shopping List:

2 ½ pound beef chuck bone-in roast
Onion

Staples/Seasonings:
Salsa, hot or medium depending on your taste
Diced tomatoes, 14 ½ ounce can
Diced green chiles, 4 ounce can
Garlic
Low sodium beef broth
Honey
Chili powder
Cumin
Salt

Roasted Garlic and Brown Sugar Pulled Roast Sandwiches

The garlic and brown sugar pair together nicely for a mouthwatering roast. You will definitely be going back for a second helping.

Ingredients:
1 (4 pound) beef pot roast, boneless
8 ounces beer
1 teaspoon salt
1 teaspoon smoked paprika
1 teaspoon pepper
1/4 cup brown sugar, lightly packed
1 teaspoon onion powder

2 heads garlic, minced or roasted

6 rolls for serving

Directions:

Place the roast on the counter and pat dry. Once dry, season with the pepper, salt, onion powder, and paprika. Place the beef into the slow cooker.

Pour the brown sugar over top of the roast and pour the beer in. Cover the slow cooker and cook on LOW for 8 hours. You can add the minced garlic, or for a special treat, you can roast the garlic. (See below.)

Remove the beef from the slow cooker and shred with a fork. If you have roasted the garlic, return the beef to the crock pot and stir in the roasted garlic. Cover and continue cooking for an additional 30 minutes. Serve on your rolls.

Roasted Garlic for a scrumptious sweet garlic taste:

Preheat the oven to 375 degrees. Cut off ¼ of the top of each garlic head off. Remove any loose paper from the garlic heads and then place the heads on a baking sheet. Pour 1 teaspoon of olive oil over top of the garlic heads and let sit for 10 minutes while the oven preheats.

Wrap the garlic in foil and place in the oven. Roast for 45 minutes. Allow the cloves to cool enough to handle and then squeeze the heads to remove the cloves. Smash the cloves of garlic with the back of a spoon.

Nutritional Information per Serving:

Servings: 6

Calories: 425

Fat: 13.4g
Carbohydrates: 8g
Protein: 64.5g

Garlic/Brown Sugar Pulled Roast Shopping List:
1 (4 pound) beef pot roast, boneless
Beer, 8 ounce bottle or can
Garlic

Staples/Seasonings:
Salt
Smoked (or regular) paprika
Pepper
Brown sugar
Onion powder
Rolls

Crock Pot Swiss Steak

Ingredients:
¼ cup flour
¼ teaspoon paprika
½ teaspoon dried thyme
Salt and pepper, to taste
2 pounds beef round steak, cut into 8 servings
1 ½ tablespoons Worcestershire sauce
1 tablespoon olive oil
1 large garlic clove, minced

2 stalks celery, sliced thin
3 cups onion, sliced
2 (14.5 ounce) cans tomatoes
½ cup beef broth

Directions:
Mix flour, paprika, and thyme in small bowl. Season as desired. Stab round steak with a fork, or pound it with a tenderizer. Brush the Worcestershire sauce over the steak. Then coat with the flour/herbs mixture.

Put olive oil in skillet. Over medium-high heat, brown steak in skillet about 5 minutes on each side. Then place the browned steak in the crock pot. Add minced garlic, celery, and sliced onions. Pour the tomatoes over the steak and vegetables.

Pour the beef stock in the skillet to loosen any leftover bits. Pour that liquid into crock pot. Cover. Cook for 8-10 hours on LOW. Cooking slower is better for this recipe, but you can also cook on HIGH for 4-5 hours if time is short.

Nutritional Information per Serving:
Serves: 8
Calories: 317
Fat: 12.2g
Carbohydrates: 12.0g
Protein: 37.9g

Swiss Steak Shopping List:
2 pounds beef round steak
Garlic cloves
Celery
Onion

Staples/Seasonings:
Flour
Paprika
Thyme
Worcestershire sauce
Olive oil
Whole tomatoes, 2 14 ½ ounce cans
Beef broth

Easy Corned Beef and Cabbage

Ingredients:
4 large red potatoes, quartered
1 pound baby carrots
1 medium onion, cut into wedges
3 cups water
3 cloves garlic, minced
1 bay leaf
2 tablespoons sugar
2 tablespoons apple cider vinegar
½ teaspoon black pepper
2 ½ pounds corned beef brisket (with spice packet)

1 head cabbage, small, cut into wedges

Directions:
Put the potatoes, carrots, and onion wedges in the bottom of the slow cooker. Mix the water, garlic, sugar, cider vinegar, pepper and the spice packet together. Pour into cooker. Add brisket and top with cabbage wedges.

Cook on LOW for 8-9 hours or until everything is tender. Discard bay leaf when finished cooking.

Nutritional Information per Serving:
Serves: 8
Calories: 547
Fat: 27.3g
Carbohydrates: 44.6g
Protein: 30.9g

Corned Beef Shopping List:
Potatoes (4 large)
Carrots (1 pound)
Onion (1 medium)
Garlic cloves
2 ½ pounds corned beef brisket (with spice packet)
1 head cabbage, small

Staples/Seasonings:
Bay leaf
Sugar
Apple Cider Vinegar

Black Pepper

Easy Pepper Steak

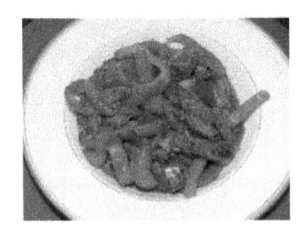

The soy sauce mixture makes the steak super tender. The soy sauce does make this recipe taste salty so you can opt for a low sodium version. If you're in a hurry, you can skip the browning in olive oil and just add the meat and garlic to the crock pot.

Ingredients: 2 tablespoons olive oil (optional, if not browning)
3 pounds beef sirloin, sliced into strips
2 cloves garlic, minced
1 onion, chopped
1/2 cup soy sauce, low sodium
2 teaspoons white sugar
1/2 teaspoon ground black pepper
2 green bell peppers, cut into strips
1 red bell pepper, cut into strips
1 tablespoon cornstarch (optional)
1/4 cup cold water (optional)

Directions:

To brown the steak, heat oil in skillet over medium heat. Add steak strips and garlic. Turn to brown on other side. Pour steak and garlic into slow cooker. Add the chopped onion, soy sauce, sugar, salt and pepper.

Cover. Cook on LOW for 6-8 hours until the beef is tender. About one hour before meal is cooked, add the peppers.

If you want to thicken the sauce, add cornstarch to water and stir into slow cooker during the last 3 minutes. Cook until the sauce thickens. Serve over brown rice or with a salad.

Nutritional information per Serving:
Serves: 6
Calories: 511
Fat: 19g
Carbohydrates: 10g
Protein: 70g

Easy Pepper Steak Shopping List:
3 pounds beef sirloin
2 cloves garlic
1 onion
2 green bell peppers
1 red bell pepper

Staples/Seasonings (if you don't have, you'll also need these):

Extra virgin olive oil
Low sodium soy sauce
White sugar
Black pepper
Cornstarch

Delicious Balsamic and Worcestershire Roast Beef

This roast smells amazing from the moment it starts cooking until it has been devoured. You will love how tender the meat is and the balsamic and Worcestershire sauce give it an irresistible taste.

Ingredients:
1 (4 pound) chuck roast, boneless
½ cup balsamic vinegar
1 cup beef broth, low sodium
1 tablespoon soy sauce
1 tablespoon Worcestershire sauce
½ teaspoon red pepper flakes
1 tablespoon honey
4 garlic cloves, minced

Directions:
Grab your roast and place it into your slow cooker. In a small bowl, whisk together the honey, vinegar, broth, Worcestershire sauce, soy sauce, garlic, and red pepper flakes until well combined.

Pour the sauce mixture over top of the roast and cover the slow cooker. Cook on HIGH for 4 hours. (If you will be gone all day, you can also cook on LOW for 6-8 hours.)

Remove the roast from the slow cooker and place on a platter. Shred with a fork and spoon ½ cup of the sauce mixture over top. Serve. (You can save the remaining gravy for another meal or use it to garnish mashed potatoes or rice.)

Nutritional Information per Serving:
Servings: 8
Calories: 511
Fat: 19g
Carbohydrates: 3.5g
Protein: 76g

Balsamic Roast Beef Shopping List:
4 pound boneless chuck roast
Garlic cloves

Staples/Seasonings:
Balsamic vinegar
Low sodium beef broth
Low sodium soy sauce
Worcestershire sauce
Red pepper flakes
Honey

Mouthwatering Beef Nachos with Fresh Pico de Gallo

These beef nachos use leftover *shredded beef* which make it a guaranteed family favorite. They also make a great game day appetizer. You and your friends will love how the flavors all come together. This party in your mouth won't stop until there are no more nachos left.

Ingredients:
2 cups leftover or freshly cooked shredded beef
1 tablespoon olive oil
1 garlic clove, minced
½ onion, chopped
8 ounces tortilla chips
2 cups black beans, in juice
2 cups shredded cheddar cheese
1 cup shredded pepper jack cheese
4 ripe avocados
1 jar salsa

Pico de Gallo:
1 (4 ounce) can diced green chilies
1 tablespoon fresh cilantro, chopped
½ onion, chopped
1 tomato, chopped

Garnish:
Guacamole
Low fat sour cream

Directions:

Sauté the garlic and onion in the olive oil in a skillet for 5 minutes. Place half of the beef mixture into your slow cooker. Next add ONE-HALF of the amounts listed above for the following ingredients in this order: tortilla chips, black beans, cheddar cheese, Pepper Jack cheese, and Pico de Gallo mixture. Repeat the layers with the rest of the main ingredients. Serve the rest of the Pico de Gallo on the side. Heat on HIGH for 1 hour until heated through.

For *quick and easy guacamole*, remove skins from 4 avocados. Remove pit and mash avocadoes in small bowl. Pour in 1/3 cup of salsa and mix thoroughly. Add more or less salsa to get the consistency you like.

Nutritional Information per Serving:
Servings: 8
Calories: 470
Fat: 17g
Carbohydrates: 44g
Protein: 37g

Beef Nachos Shopping List:
Leftover shredded beef or see Shredded Beef Recipe for that shopping list
Garlic
Onion
Tortilla chips

Cheddar cheese (1 package)
Pepper jack cheese (1 package)
Diced green chiles (1 4 ounce can)
Cilantro, 1 bunch fresh
1 tomato
4 ripe avocados
1 jar salsa
Low fat sour cream

Staples/Seasonings:
Olive oil
Black beans

Roast Beef with Pineapple

Ingredients:
1 (8 ounce) can unsweetened sliced pineapple
3 pounds beef top round roast, cut in half
¼ cup flour
1 teaspoon salt
¼ teaspoon pepper
1 medium onion, sliced
¼ teaspoon ground ginger
¼ cup brown sugar
2 tablespoons cornstarch
½ teaspoon minced garlic
½ cup beef broth
¼ cup soy sauce, low-sodium

1 green pepper, sliced

Directions:

Drain pineapple and reserve the juice. Refrigerate the pineapple to use later. Mix flour, pepper, and salt and rub into roast. Lay sliced onion in bottom of slow cooker. Add roast. Combine ginger, brown sugar, cornstarch, and garlic. Stir in the beef broth, soy sauce, and reserved pineapple juice. Pour sauce over the meat. Cover and cook on LOW for 6-7 hours.

Add sliced pineapple and green pepper. Cook 1 hour more or until meat is tender.

Nutritional Information per Serving:
Serves: 10
Calories: 211
Fat: 6.0g
Carbohydrates: 14.6g
Protein: 26.6g

Pineapple Roast Beef Shopping List:
1 (8 ounce) can unsweetened sliced pineapple
3 pounds beef top round roast
1 onion
1 green pepper

Staples/Seasonings:
Flour
Salt

Pepper
Ginger
Brown sugar
Cornstarch
Beef Broth
Low sodium soy sauce
Garlic

Slow Cooker Cheeseburgers

Everyone loves a delicious cheeseburger and these slow cooked burgers are the best of the best. They are easy to make and you can enjoy them any time of the year even if you don't have a grill.

Ingredients:
1 tablespoon olive oil
3 pounds ground beef, 93% lean
½ teaspoon pepper
½ teaspoon salt
1 sweet onion, chopped
6 ounces shredded cheddar cheese
3 tablespoons milk
2 garlic cloves, minced
3 tablespoons mustard
3 tablespoons ketchup

Toppings:

Tomatoes, lettuce, sliced onions, sliced tomatoes, avocado, buns

Directions:
(This recipe takes a little longer prep because you cook the ground beef prior to adding everything in the slow cooker. To save time, you can cook the lean ground beef and freeze and then take out of freezer and use. The benefit is that this recipe is done in just a few hours...perfect for weekends!)

Grab a large skillet and place it over medium high heat. Add in the olive oil and allow to heat. Once hot, add in the onions. Cook for 3 minutes and then stir in the garlic. Cook for 30 seconds.
Add the beef to the skillet and season with salt and pepper. Stir well and cook until the meat is browned, about 5 minutes.

Place the beef in the slow cooker and add in the ketchup, milk, and mustard. Stir well. Add in the cheese and stir again. Cover and cook on LOW for 3-4 hours making sure to stir every 30 seconds. Serve with buns and additional toppings.

Nutritional Information per Serving:
Servings: 8
Calories: 452
Fat: 20g
Carbohydrates: 5g

Protein: 58g

Slow Cooker Cheeseburger Shopping List:
3 pounds lean ground beef
1 sweet onion
6 ounces cheddar cheese (or your favorite cheese)
Low fat milk
Garlic

Staples/Seasonings:
Olive oil
Pepper
Salt
Mustard
Ketchup

Tender Coconut Curry Vegetables and Beef

This is a hearty meal that will delight the whole family. It is a combination of sweet and mildly spicy flavors that will take your taste buds on a journey across the world with every bite.

Ingredients:
2 pounds beef chuck roast
2 tablespoons olive or vegetable oil
1 teaspoon salt
4 garlic cloves, minced
1 large onion, cut into wedges
1 tablespoon ground ginger

2 teaspoons soy sauce

1 tablespoon brown sugar, packed

1 (12 ounce) can coconut milk, light

1 tablespoon curry powder

1/2 teaspoon cayenne pepper

1 yellow bell pepper, chopped

1 pint cherry tomatoes

Directions:

Place beef on a clean surface and pat dry. Chop into 2 inch chunks and then season with salt.

In a large skillet over medium high heat, allow oil to warm and then add in the beef. Cook until beef is browned evenly on all sides, 8-10 minutes.

Place the beef in your crock pot and add in the garlic, onions, soy sauce, and ginger. In a small bowl, whisk together the brown sugar, coconut milk, cayenne pepper, and curry powder until blended. Pour over top of the beef.

Cover and cook on LOW for 4-5 hours. During the last 15 minutes of cook time, add in the bell pepper and tomatoes. Stir and continue cooking for the remaining 15 minutes. Serve.

Nutritional Information per Serving:

Servings: 6

Calories: 450

Fat: 35g

Carbohydrates: 15g
Protein: 35g

Coconut Curry Beef Shopping List:
2 pounds beef chuck roast
1 yellow bell pepper
1 (12 ounce) can coconut milk, light
1 pint cherry tomatoes
4 garlic cloves
1 large onion

Staples/Seasonings:
Olive or vegetable oil
Ginger
Salt
Low sodium soy sauce
Curry powder
Brown sugar
Cayenne pepper

Easy Slow Cooker Meatballs

Ingredients:
1 cup low-fat milk
¾ cup quick-cooking oats
3 tablespoons onion, finely chopped
1 ½ teaspoons salt
1 ½ pounds lean ground beef

1 cup ketchup
½ cup water
3 tablespoons apple cider vinegar
2 tablespoons sugar

Directions:
Combine milk, oats, onion, and salt, mixing well. Then add ground beef and mix all ingredients well. Shape into 1 inch balls and lay in crock pot.

Combine the last four ingredients in a small bowl. Stir well and add to crock pot over meatballs. Cover. Cook for 7-8 hours on LOW or until meat is cooked through.

Nutritional Information per Serving:
Serves: 6
Calories: 324
Fat: 8.2g
Carbohydrates: 23.6g
Protein: 37.9g

Meatballs Shopping List:
1 cup low fat milk
Oatmeal, quick cooking
Onion
1 ½ pounds lean ground beef

Staples/Seasonings:
Salt
Ketchup

Apple cider vinegar

Sugar

Lighter Beef and Mushroom Stroganoff

Who doesn't love a home cooked stroganoff? Now you can enjoy the delicious flavors without slaving away all day in the kitchen.

Ingredients:

1 1/2 pounds beef chuck steak

1/2 cup white wine

2 tablespoons tomato sauce

1 cup beef broth, low sodium

1 pound mushrooms, sliced

2 small onions, chopped

4 tablespoons soy sauce, low sodium

1/4 teaspoon pepper

1 cup sour cream, reduced fat

2 tablespoons cornstarch

Directions:

Place your beef on a clean surface and trim off any excess fat. Once trimmed, pat dry and chop into 2 inch cubes. Place the beef in the crock pot. Add in the wine, tomato sauce, broth, mushrooms, onions, and 3 tablespoons of the soy sauce.

Cover and cook on HIGH for 4 hours. (You can also cook on LOW for 6 hours.)

In a small mixing bowl, whisk together the remaining soy sauce, pepper, sour cream, and cornstarch until well blended. Slowly add into the crock pot and whisk. Continue cooking an additional 30 minutes or until the sauce is thick. Serve over egg noodles or pasta.

Nutritional Information per Serving:
Servings: 6
Calories: 246
Fat: 8g
Carbohydrates: 1g
Protein: 26g

Beef Stroganoff Shopping List:
1 1/2 pounds beef chuck steak
2 onions
1 pound mushrooms
White wine
Sour cream, reduced fat

Staples/Seasonings:
Beef broth, low sodium preferred
Pepper
Cornstarch
Tomato sauce
Soy sauce, low sodium

CHICKEN RECIPES

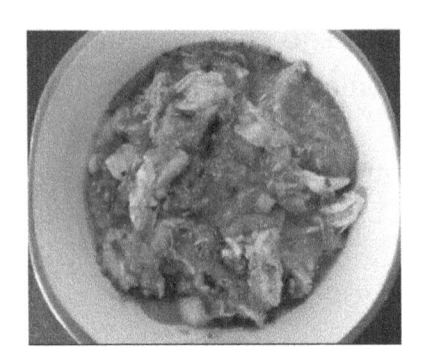

Slow Cooked Lime and Cilantro Chicken

This delicious chicken is one of our family's favorites. The cilantro and lime cook to create delicious flavor to create a sassy meal. You can serve this dish with rice or even place the chicken on some tortillas, yum.

Ingredients:
3 pounds boneless, skinless chicken breast halves
1/2 (1 1/4 ounce) package taco seasoning mix
1 (16 ounce) jar salsa
3 tablespoons fresh cilantro, chopped
1 lime, juiced

Directions:

Add the taco seasoning and salsa to your slow cooker. Stir well. Add in the chicken breasts and press down to cover with the liquid. Cover and cook on HIGH for 4 hours. (You can also cook on LOW for 6-8 hours.)

About an hour before finished, add the cilantro and the lime. Before serving, shred the chicken.

Nutritional Information per Serving:
Servings: 6
Calories: 272
Fat: 4.7g
Carbohydrates: 9.3g
Protein: 45.3g

Lime and Cilantro Chicken Shopping List:
3 pounds boneless, skinless chicken breast halves
Fresh cilantro
1 lime

Staples/Seasonings:
Taco seasoning mix
1 (16 ounce) jar salsa

Crock Pot Lemon Chicken with Baby Carrots

Nothing pairs together as nicely as chicken and lemon. This chicken is delicately flavored with a lemon flavor that will keep you happy bite after bite.

Ingredients:
8 boneless, skinless chicken thighs, chopped into 1 inch pieces
1/3 cup flour
1 teaspoon salt
1/8 teaspoon pepper
2 tablespoons butter
1 bag baby carrots
1 onion, chopped
3 garlic cloves, minced
¼ cup lemon juice
1 teaspoon dried oregano
1 cup chicken broth, low sodium
1 tablespoon brown sugar
1 tablespoon cornstarch
¼ cup water

Directions:
Place the flour, salt, and pepper in a small bowl and toss. Dredge the chicken in the flour mixture and then shake off the excess flour. Place the butter in a large skillet and allow to melt. Once melted, brown the chicken in the skillet for 3 minutes.

In your slow cooker, place the carrots, onion, and garlic along the bottom. Place the chicken on top. Add the lemon juice, oregano, chicken broth, and brown sugar to the skillet the chicken was in. Continue cooking making sure to scrape up the browned bits to include in this mixture. Let this reach a boil and then pour over top of the chicken in the crock pot.

Cover the crock pot and cook on LOW for 7-8 hours. (You can also cook on HIGH for 3-4 hours.) Right before serving, whisk the water and cornstarch together until blended. Stir this into the crock pot. Cook for another 30 minutes on HIGH and then serve.

Nutritional Information per Serving:
Servings: 4
Calories: 400
Fat: 13g
Carbohydrates: 18g
Protein: 50g

Lemon Chicken Shopping List:
8 boneless, skinless chicken thighs
1 bag baby carrots
1 onion
3 garlic cloves
3-4 lemons

Staples/Seasonings:
Flour

Salt
Pepper
Butter
Oregano, dried
Chicken broth, low sodium
Brown sugar
Cornstarch

Crock Pot Marinara Vegetables with Chicken

This is the perfect slow cooked meal for any day of the week. Not only is it easy to make, it is super delicious.

Ingredients:
2 pounds boneless, skinless chicken breasts
4 tomatoes, chopped
4 garlic cloves, peeled and then crushed
1 jar (18 ounces) marinara sauce, low sodium
1 cup celery ribs, chopped
1 green bell pepper, core and seeds removed, chopped
2 cups zucchini, chopped
1 teaspoon dried thyme
1 teaspoon dried basil

Directions:
Place all of the chicken into the crock pot. Add the tomatoes, garlic, zucchini, celery, and pepper. Pour the

marinara sauce into the crock pot and then top with the thyme and basil.

Cover and cook on LOW for 6 to 7 hours. Remove the chicken and shred. Return the chicken to the crock pot and stir. Serve.

Nutritional Information per Serving:
Servings: 8
Calories: 176.8
Fat: 3.7g
Carbohydrates: 7.9g
Protein: 26.8g

Marinara Vegetables with Chicken Shopping List:
2 pounds boneless, skinless chicken breasts
4 tomatoes
4 garlic cloves
Celery
1 green bell pepper
2-3 zucchini

Staples/Seasonings:
1 jar (18 ounces) marinara sauce, low sodium
Thyme
Basil

Tender Herbed Chicken

The fresh herbs and wine in this recipe create an inviting, delicious meal. If you have children, don't worry about the wine. The alcohol in the wine cooks out in the cooking process, leaving a fall-apart tasty meal.

Ingredients:
1 teaspoon extra virgin olive oil
4 chicken breasts, skinless (about 1 ½ pounds)
1/2 teaspoon Himalayan or Kosher salt
1/4 teaspoon black pepper
1 medium onion, peeled and diced
5 cloves garlic, peeled and minced
1 tablespoon fresh rosemary, chopped (or 1 teaspoon dried)
1 tablespoon fresh thyme, chopped (or 1 teaspoon dried)
1 tablespoon fresh oregano, chopped (or 1 teaspoon dried)
1 cup white wine
3/4 cup chicken broth, low sodium
1/3 cup all-purpose flour
Salt and pepper to taste

Directions:
Heat olive oil in a large skillet, using medium-high heat. Season the chicken breasts with the salt and pepper and lay in skillet. Sear for 2 to 3 minutes per side (or until lightly golden).

Pour the chopped onions, garlic, and herbs into the crock pot. Lay the chicken breast over the garlic and herb layer. Combine the low sodium broth, white wine, and flour in a bowl, stirring until the flour is completely mixed in. Pour the wine mixture over the chicken.

Cover and set your crock pot for 4 hours on HIGH (or if you'll be gone all day, you can set it for 8 hours on LOW). Serve with a fresh green salad, or your favorite grains – brown rice, couscous, or pasta, brown rice.

Nutritional Information per Serving:
Serves: 4
Calories: 453
Fat: 14.4g
Carbohydrates: 15.3g
Protein: 51.9g

Herbed Chicken Shopping List:
4 chicken breasts, skinless (about 1 ½ pounds)
1 medium onion
5 cloves garlic
Fresh rosemary
Fresh thyme
Fresh oregano
White wine

Staples/Seasonings:
Olive oil
Himalayan or Kosher salt
Pepper, black
Chicken broth, low sodium
Flour

Salt
Dried rosemary, if fresh not available
Dried thyme, if fresh not available
Dried oregano, if fresh not available

Sweet Potato, Mushroom, and Chicken Stew

Ingredients:
6 chicken thighs, bone-in, skin removed, trimmed of fat
2 pounds sweet potatoes, peeled and cut into spears
½ pound mushrooms, white button, thinly sliced
6 large shallots, peeled and halved
4 cloves garlic, peeled, minced
1 cup dry white wine
2 teaspoons chopped fresh rosemary (or ½ teaspoon dried rosemary, crushed)
1 teaspoon salt
½ teaspoon black pepper
1 ½ tablespoons wine vinegar, white

Directions:
Set aside the white-wine vinegar. Put all the other ingredients into a 6-quart crock pot. Stir. Cover. Cook on LOW for 5-6 hours, until potatoes are soft. If preferred, remove chicken meat from bones once done. Stir in wine vinegar. Serve.

Nutritional Information per Serving:

Serves: 6
Calories: 285
Fat: 6g
Carbohydrates: 35g
Protein: 17g

Chicken Stew Shopping List:
6 chicken thighs, bone-in
2 pounds sweet potatoes
½ pound mushrooms, white button
6 large shallots
4 cloves garlic
White wine
Fresh rosemary

Staples/Seasonings:
Dried rosemary, if fresh not available
Salt
Pepper, black
White wine vinegar

Cashew Chicken

Ingredients:
2 pounds boneless, skinless chicken breasts (about 4 pieces), cut into smaller pieces
1/4 cup all purpose flour
1/2 tsp black pepper

1 tablespoon extra virgin olive oil
1/4 cup soy sauce
2 tablespoon rice vinegar
2 tablespoon ketchup
1 tablespoon brown sugar
1 garlic clove, minced
1/2 tsp grated fresh ginger
1/4 tsp red pepper flakes
1/2 cup raw cashews
Instant brown rice

Directions:
Pour flour and pepper into gallon food storage bag. Cut chicken into small pieces. Add to bag and shake to coat. Grab a large skillet, add olive oil and heat over medium high heat. Add coated chicken; brown for about 2 minutes on each side. Add chicken to the crock pot. .

In a small bowl, mix together all the remaining ingredients except the cashews. Pour over chicken. Cook on LOW for 4 hours. Add cashews, stir, and serve over cooked brown rice. (Instant brown rice is a time saver!)

Nutritional Information per Serving:
Serves: 6
Calories: 413
Fat: 18.9g
Carbohydrates: 11.7g
Protein: 46.9g

Cashew Chicken Shopping List:

2 pounds boneless, skinless chicken breasts (about 4 pieces), cut into smaller pieces

Garlic

Ginger

Raw cashew, ½ cup

Staples/Seasonings:

Flour

Pepper, black

Olive oil

Soy sauce

Rice vinegar

Ketchup

Brown sugar

Red pepper flakes

Instant/quick-cooking brown rice

Crock Pot Wild Rice and Chicken Stew

This stew is very hearty and extremely delicious. Serve it with some bread and you have a complete meal that will satisfy and warm everyone.

Ingredients:

4 boneless, skinless chicken breasts

1 cup wild rice, uncooked, rinsed, and drained

1 medium onion, chopped

3 celery stalks, chopped
3 carrots, peeled and diced
2 bay leaves
2 garlic cloves, minced
½ teaspoon dried thyme
6 cups chicken broth, low sodium
¼ cup parsley, chopped
Salt and pepper, to taste

Directions:
Place the carrots, onions, garlic, celery, bay leaves, thyme, pepper, and rice into the crock pot. Place the chicken breasts on top and then pour the chicken broth over top. Cover the crock pot and cook on LOW for 6 to 6 ½ hours. (You can also cook on HIGH for 3 ½ hours)

Remove the chicken from the slow cooker and shred with a fork. Return the chicken to the crock pot and stir. Remove and discard the bay leaves. Add in the parsley and serve. Season with additional salt and pepper if needed.

Nutritional Information per Serving:
Servings: 8
Calories: 300
Fat: 10g
Carbohydrates: 25g
Protein: 35g

Rice and Chicken Stew Shopping List:

4 boneless, skinless chicken breasts
1 cup wild rice
1 medium onion
Celery
Carrots
Garlic
Parsley

Staples/Seasonings:
Bay leaves
Dried thyme
Chicken broth, low sodium
Salt
Pepper, black

Slow Cooker Taco Soup with Chicken

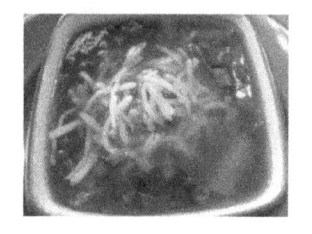

Surprisingly after cooking all day, the corn is still crisp and not soggy. The flavors with the beer and seasonings are absolutely wonderful!

Ingredients:
3 boneless, skinless chicken breasts

1 (12 ounce) can beer
1 (8 ounce) can tomato sauce
1 (14 1/2 ounce) can diced tomatoes
1 (14 1/2 ounce) can black beans
1 (16 ounce) can chili beans
1 (15 ounce) can whole kernel corn, drained
1 (4 ounce) can diced green chiles
1 onion, chopped
1/2 packet (1 1/4 ounces) taco seasoning

Optional Toppings:
Shredded mozzarella cheese
Tortilla chips (try blue corn chips for a great taste)
Low-fat sour cream

Directions:
Place the beer, tomato sauce, tomatoes, black beans, chili beans, corn, green chiles, and onion in your slow cooker. Stir well. Add in the taco seasoning and stir well to evenly distribute.

Place the chicken breasts on top and lightly press down to cover them with the mixture. Cover and cook on LOW for 5 hours.

Remove the chicken and shred with a fork. Return the chicken to the slow cooker and continue cooking for an additional 2 hours. Serve.

Nutritional Information per Serving:

Servings: 8
Calories: 434
Fat: 17.7g
Carbohydrates: 42.3g
Protein: 27.2g

Chicken Taco Soup Shopping List:
3 boneless, skinless chicken breasts
1 onion
1 (12 ounce) can beer
1 (16 ounce) can chili beans

Staples/Seasonings:
1 (15 ounce) can whole kernel corn, drained
1 (8 ounce) can tomato sauce
1 (14 1/2 ounce) can black beans
1 (14 1/2 ounce) can diced tomatoes
1 (4 ounce) can diced green chiles
1/2 packet (1 1/4 ounces) taco seasoning

Crock Pot Creamy Chicken Stroganoff

This is a play on traditional beef stroganoff. This recipe is perfect for anyone who loves chicken. The sauce is creamy and dreamy and uses canned soup and dressing mixes for those days when you're running late!

Ingredients:
4 boneless, skinless chicken breast halves, chopped

1 (.7 ounce) package Italian style salad dressing mix, dried
1/8 cup butter
1 (8 ounce) package reduced fat cream cheese
1 (10 ¾ ounce) can condensed cream of chicken soup, low sodium

Directions:
Place the chicken, dressing, and butter into your crock pot and stir. Cover and cook on LOW for 5-6 hours. Stir the soup and cream cheese into the crock pot and mix well. Cook for an additional 30 minutes.

Serve over egg noodles or pasta. If you are eating less gluten, try gluten-free pasta or brown rice.

Nutritional Information per Serving:
Servings: 4
Calories: 456
Fat: 31g
Carbohydrates: 9.5g
Protein: 33.4g

Chicken Stroganoff Shopping List:
4 boneless, skinless chicken breast halves
Butter
1 (8 ounce) package reduced fat cream cheese

Staples/Seasonings:
1 (.7 ounce) package Italian style salad dressing mix, dried

1 (10 ¾ ounce) can condensed low-sodium cream of chicken soup

Cheesy Slow Cooker Chicken & Rice

Ingredients:

1 pound boneless skinless chicken breasts
½ cup onion, chopped
1 (10.5 ounce) can cream of chicken soup, low-fat type
1 (8 ounce) package boxed Zatarain's brand New Orleans Rice
1 cup Mexican cheese blend or Cheddar Cheese
1 (15 ounce) can kernel corn, drained

Directions:
Place the chicken breasts in the bottom of the crock pot. Mix the chopped onion and the cream soup and pour over chicken. Cook for 7-8 hours on LOW (or alternatively, you can cook this on HIGH for 3-4 hours).

Just before the chicken is finished cooking, prepare the rice according to package directions. Mix the rice with the Mexican cheese and the corn. Add to the crock pot and stir. Cook for another 10-15 minutes until everything is heated through and the cheese has melted.

Nutritional Information per Serving:

Serves: 6
Calories: 452
Fat: 15.2g
Carbohydrates: 47g
Protein: 32.3g

Cheesy Chicken and Rice Shopping List:

1 pound boneless skinless chicken breasts

Onion

1 (8 ounce) package boxed Zatarain's brand New Orleans Rice

Shredded Mexican cheese blend or Cheddar Cheese

Staples/Seasonings:

1 (10.5 ounce) can cream of chicken soup, low-fat type

1 (15 ounce) can kernel corn, drained

Juicy Crock Pot Chicken Marbella

This dish is the perfect dinner any night of the week. Your home will be delightfully filled with the scent of the chicken slow-cooking all day.

Ingredients:

4 chicken drumsticks and 4 thighs with skin removed

2 tablespoons brown sugar

1/2 cup dry white wine

1 1/2 teaspoons dried oregano

Salt and pepper, to taste

3 tablespoons red wine vinegar

1 tablespoon capers

6 garlic cloves, minced

1/4 cup green olives, pitted

1/2 cup prunes

1/4 cup fresh parsley, chopped
1 cup long grain rice

Directions:
Place the brown sugar, wine, salt, pepper, oregano, and 2 tablespoons of the vinegar in your slow cooker. Whisk together until combined. Add in the capers, garlic, olives, and prunes. Mix well.

Place the chicken on top and lightly press down to submerge in the mixture. Cover and cook on LOW for 5-6 hours. (Alternatively, you can cook on HIGH for 3 to 4 hours.) Stir in the remaining vinegar and parsley.

Cook the rice according to the direction on the package 30 minutes before the dish is done. Serve.

Nutritional Information per Serving:
Servings: 4
Calories: 302
Fat: 8g
Carbohydrates: 32g
Protein: 34g

Chicken Marbella Shopping List:
4 chicken drumsticks and 4 thighs
White wine
Capers
Garlic

Green olives
Prunes
Fresh parsley

Staples/Seasonings:
Brown sugar
Dried oregano
Red wine vinegar
Long grain rice
Salt
Pepper, black

Garlic and Cinnamon Slow Cooked Chicken

This is the perfect dish for any family event or even just a nice dinner. The cinnamon and garlic provide a nice taste to the chicken and you can smell this slow cook all day long. Your first bite will already have you thinking about seconds.

Ingredients:
1 (5 pound) roasting chicken
1 tablespoon olive oil
1 tablespoon butter, unsalted
2 cinnamon sticks
8 garlic cloves, minced
2 oranges, zested
2 cups milk, 2% (or low fat)
1 teaspoon dried thyme
Salt and pepper, to taste

Directions:

Place the chicken on a clean surface and season it with a liberal amount of salt and pepper. Place the oil and butter in a large skillet and allow to melt. Once melted, add in the chicken and brown on both sides, about 8 minutes. Place the chicken in the slow cooker with the breast side down.

Reserve 2 teaspoons of the oil and butter from the pan and drain the rest. Add the cinnamon, and garlic to the pan and cook for 2 minutes. Pour into the slow cooker.

Add the orange zest, milk, and thyme to the slow cooker and stir well. Cover and cook on HIGH for 4 hours. (You can also cook on LOW for 6 hours.) Serve.

Nutritional Information per Serving:
Servings: 8
Calories: 194
Fat: 8.7g
Carbohydrates: 9.9g
Protein: 19.1g

Garlic and Cinnamon Chicken Shopping List:
1 (5 pound) roasting chicken
2 cups milk, 2%
Unsalted butter
2 oranges
Garlic

Staples/Seasonings:
Olive oil
Cinnamon sticks
Dried thyme
Salt
Pepper, black

Spicy Chorizo Chicken

This is a hearty Mexican style meal. The chorizo sausage ups the fat content, but the flavors of the chicken with the sausage and spices are simply delicious.

Ingredients:
1 ½ pounds boneless, skinless chicken breast halves
1 onion, chopped
1 (10 ounce) can tomato sauce
1 (7 ounce) can chipotle chili peppers in adobo sauce
2 fresh jalapeno peppers
1 cloves garlic, minced
1 teaspoon ground oregano
1 teaspoon ground cumin
1 teaspoon chili powder
¼ teaspoon red pepper flakes
¾ pound chorizo sausage

Directions:
Remove seeds from chili peppers and jalapeno peppers. Chop peppers. Combine with remaining ingredients

(except chorizo sausage). Stir together and cook on LOW for 2 ½ to 3 hours. Take two forks, remove chicken from crock pot, and shred. Return to cooker.

Cook the chorizo sausage in a large skillet over medium-high heat, until thoroughly cooked and crumbly. This will take 5-10 minutes. Drain. Freeze grease and discard. Stir cooked chorizo into chicken mixture. Cook on LOW for 1 more hour.

Serve with garlic bread or corn bread.

Nutritional Information per Serving:
Serves: 8
Calories: 337
Fat: 19.6g
Carbohydrates: 5.0g
Protein: 34.6g

Chorizo Chicken Shopping List:
1 ½ pounds boneless, skinless chicken breast halves
1 onion
1 (7 ounce) can chipotle chili peppers in adobo sauce
2 fresh jalapeno peppers
Garlic
¾ pound chorizo sausage

Staples/Seasonings:
1 (10 ounce) can tomato sauce
Dried oregano

Ground cumin
Chili powder
Red pepper flakes

Slow Cooker Chicken and Dumplings

This recipe uses several pre-made items, but kids love this recipe, so we had to include this one! It reminds us of grandma's homemade chicken and dumplings recipe – only this one is super simple.

Ingredients:
4 boneless, skinless chicken breast halves (about 1 ½ pounds)
1 tablespoons butter (optional)
1 onion, chopped
2 (10 ¾ ounce) cans reduced fat condensed cream of chicken soup
1 (10 ounce) package refrigerated biscuits, torn
1 ½ to 2 cups water (or enough to cover the chicken)

Directions:
Place the butter, chicken, onion, and soup into the slow cooker. Add just enough water to cover the mixture. Cover and cook on HIGH for 5-6 hours.
Toss in the biscuits 30 minutes before the cook time is up. Serve.

Nutritional Information per Serving:

Servings: 8
Calories: 299
Fat: 11g
Carbohydrates: 20.9g
Protein: 27.5g

Chicken and Dumplings Shopping List:
4 boneless, skinless chicken breast halves
1 (10 ounce) package refrigerated biscuits, torn
1 onion
Butter

Staples/Seasonings:
2 (10 ¾ ounce) cans reduced fat condensed cream of chicken soup

Delicious Mexican Chicken Tortilla Soup

This is a delicious Mexican meal that will add a bit of flare and spice to your dinner table. This recipe is easy to make and will delight the whole family. Serve with some white or brown rice or warm tortillas to complete the whole meal.

Ingredients:
1 pound chicken, cooked and shredded
1 (4 ounce) can green chili peppers, chopped
1 (15 ounce) can whole peeled tomatoes, crushed

1 (10 ounce) can enchilada sauce
2 garlic cloves, minced
1 onion, chopped
1 (14 1/2 ounce) can chicken broth, low sodium
1 cups water
1 teaspoon chili powder
1 teaspoon salt
1 teaspoon cumin
1/4 teaspoon pepper
1 bay leaf
2 tablespoon fresh cilantro, chopped
1 (10 ounce) package frozen corn
7 corn tortillas
Whipped butter or soft margarine

Directions:
Place the green chilies, tomatoes, enchilada sauce, garlic, onion, and chicken into your slow cooker. Add in the chicken broth, water, chili powder, salt, cumin, pepper, and bay leaf. Stir well. Stir in the cilantro and corn and cover.
Cook on LOW for 6-8 hours. (You can also cook on HIGH for 3-4 hours.)
Preheat your oven to 400 degrees Fahrenheit. Place the tortillas on a baking sheet and lightly brush with butter or margarine. Cook in the oven for 15 minutes until crisp. Chop and sprinkle over top of the soup. Serve.

Nutritional Information per Serving:
Servings: 8

Calories: 262
Fat: 10.8g
Carbohydrates: 24.7g
Protein: 18g

Chicken Tortilla Soup Shopping List:
1 pound chicken, cooked and shredded (buy a roasted chicken to make it easier)
1 (15 ounce) can whole peeled tomatoes, crushed
1 (4 ounce) can green chili peppers, chopped
1 (10 ounce) can enchilada sauce
1 onion
Garlic
7 corn tortillas
Fresh cilantro
Whipped butter or soft margarine

Staples/Seasonings:
1 (4 ounce) can green chili peppers, chopped
1 (10 ounce) package frozen corn
1 (14 1/2 ounce) can chicken broth, low sodium
Chili powder
Salt
Cumin
Pepper, black
Bay leaf

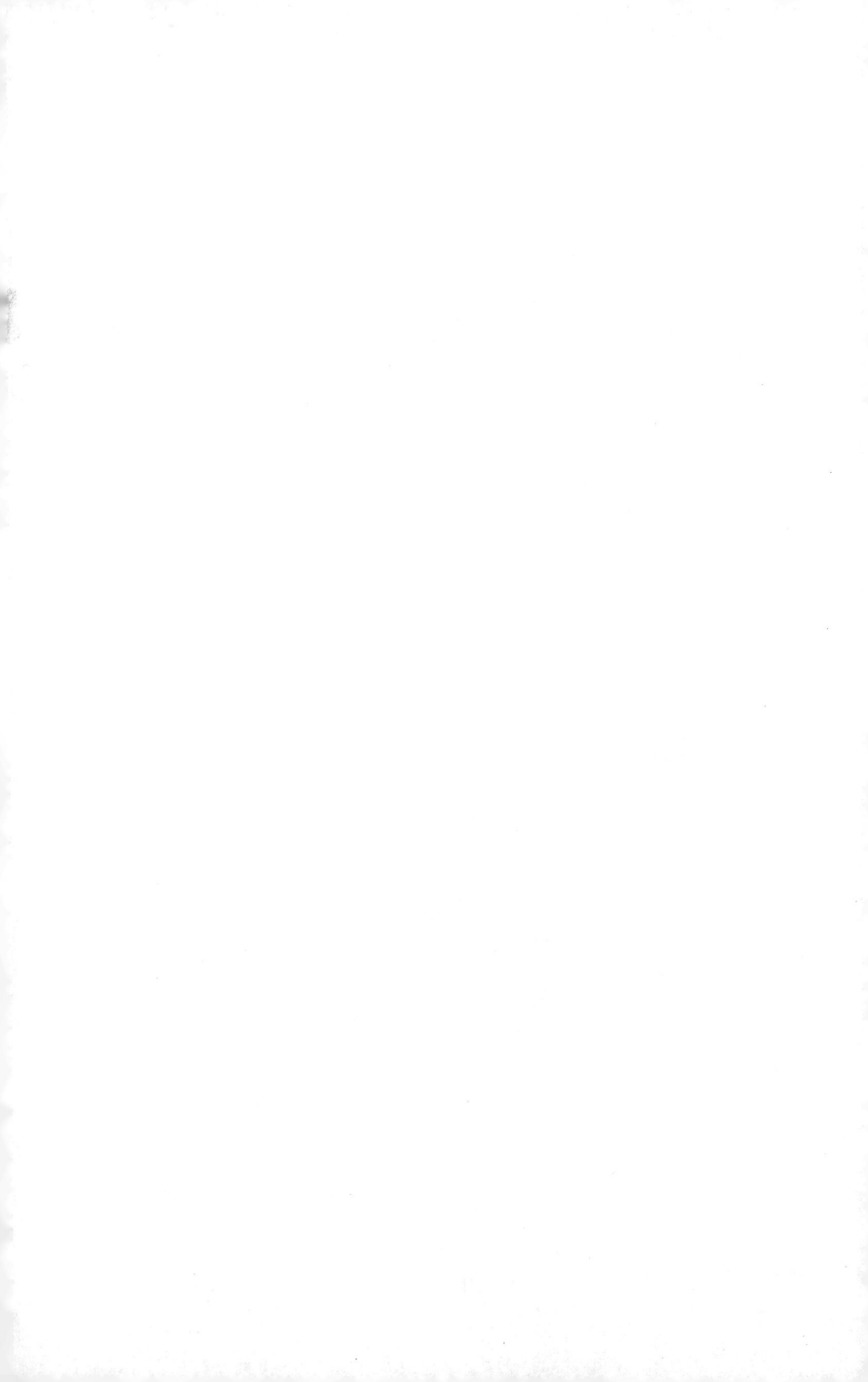